#MANUP

CW00544462

TOUGH
T TALK

ALSO PUBLISHED BY DAWN PUBLISHING

The Relentless Rebel Duology by Dawn Bates:

Friday Bridge – Becoming a Muslim; becoming everyone's business

(1st Edition, 2013; 2nd Edition, 2017; 3rd Edition, 2023)

Walaahi – A Firsthand Account of Living Through The Egyptian Uprising And Why I Walked Away From Islaam (1st Edition, 2017; 2nd Edition 2023)

Anthologies:

Break Down to Wake Up – Journey Beyond the Now by Jocelyn Bellows (2020)

Standing in Strength – Inspirational Stories of Power Unleashed by Laarni Mulvey (2021)

The Potent Power of Menopause – A Culturally Diverse Perspective of Feminine Transformation by Dawn Bates and Clarissa Kristjansson (2022)

Alive to Thrive – Life After Attempting Suicide: Our Stories by Dawn Bates and Debbie Debonaire (2022)

Memoirs/Biographies:

Crossing The Line – A Journey of Purpose and Self-Belief by Dawn Bates (2017)

Becoming Annie – The Biography of a Curious Woman by Dawn Bates (2020)

Becoming the Champion – V1 Awareness by Korey Carpenter (2020)

Unlocked – Discovering Your Hidden Keys by Carmelle Crinnion (2020)

The Recipe – A US Marine's Mindset to Success by Jake Cosme (2021)

Continued…

Skills Development:

51 Powerful Ps of Public Speaking by Krystylle L Richardson (2022)

The Sacral Series by Dawn Bates:

Moana – One Woman's Journey Back to Self (2020)

Leila – A Life Renewed One Canvas at a Time (2020)

Pandora – Melting the Ice One Dive at a Time (2021)

Alpha – Saving Humanity One Vagina at a Time (2021)

The Democ-Chu Series by Nath Brye:

Slave Boy (2020)

Blood Child (2021)

Sin Eater – Memories Vanish When She Appears by Amanda Denham (2024)

Are you a writer?

Do you want to get published?

Then visit https://dawnbates.com/writers and see how we can help you on your journey to getting published!

To discover the latest Dawn Publishing books, please visit https://dawnbates.com/readers

#MANUP

Reducing male suicide and destroying the stigma one story at a time

TOUGH T TALK

Curated by Steve Whittle
Founder of Tough to Talk Charity

© 2024 Dawn Bates

Published by Dawn Publishing

www.dawnbates.com

The moral right of the authors has been asserted.

Cataloguing-in-Publication entry is available from the British Library.

ISBN : 978-1-913973-39-1 (paperback)

978-1-913973-45-2 (hardback)

978-1-913973-40-7 (ebook)

Book cover design: Jerry Lampson

All rights reserved. No part of this book may be reproduced, stored in a retrieval system, communicated or transmitted in any form or by means without written permission. All inquiries should be made to the publisher at the above address.

Disclaimer: The material in this publication is of the nature of general comment only and does not represent professional advice. It is not intended to provide specific guidance for particular circumstances and should not be relied on as the basis for any decision to take action or not to take action on any matters which it covers.

The opinions expressed in this publication are those of the contributors and do not reflect the opinions of Dawn Publishing, Dawn Bates International, its Editors, or Tough To Talk.

Information contained within this book has been obtained by Dawn Publishing from sources believed to be reliable. However, neither Dawn Publishing, Dawn Bates International Ltd or Tough To Talk guarantees the accuracy or completeness of any information published herein and neither Dawn Publishing, Dawn Bates International Ltd, its Editors or Tough To Talk shall be responsible for any errors, omissions, or claims for damages, including exemplary damages, arising out of use, inability to use, or with regard to the accuracy or sufficiency of the information contained within.

Neither the editor, authors, publisher, or any other party associated with the production of ManUp Tough To Talk accept responsibility for any accident or injury resulting from reading the content contained herein. Any individual choosing to select, purchase and read this book does so at their own risk, and must take full responsibility for their own choices, health and well-being.

*This book is dedicated to the courageous men who,
in their journey to #MANUP,
found their true masculinity in the heart of vulnerability.*

THIS IS ME

In depths of life's grand tale behold
A man named Steve, his story to be told
Ex Royal Navy, I sailed the seas
Where wild adventures filled my soul with ease.
Half my days in exotic lands I spent,
where spirits flowed and merriment was meant.
The other half with thunderous sound,
I blew things up on battlegrounds renowned.
Now I dance in events' embrace,
and project management, joyful pace.
With jazz hands high I spread the light,
infusing every moment with fun and light.
In love's embrace I found bliss –
A wonderful girlfriend and kids I could miss.
An amazing pooch, loyal and true,
my heart content, a love that grew.
A circle of friends, small and strong,
trustworthy souls where I belong.
A charity founder, a noble quest –
supporting lives with love addressed.
Business and communities I will mend,
With care and kindness my soul to lend.
So when asked how I'm doing, you'll hear me say
"I'm top banana, brightening each day".
My life is wonderful, a song to sing,
through every twist, through everything.
This is me, I proudly proclaim –
In my story, a legacy ingrained.

THIS IS ALSO ME

In the depths of my soul, a secret hides —
A world within me where darkness resides.
This is also me, concealed every day,
Behind a mask of strength on stoic display.
Complex PTSD echoes through my core,
Leaving scars unseen, wounds too deep to ignore.
Add a companion that walks by my side,
A restless mind dancing, unable to abide
Depression's embrace, a heavy weight I bear,
Casting shadows upon me, an endless affair.
Thoughts of suicide — they haunt me at night.
A constant companion. A treacherous fight.
Three times I faced the edge, teetering there,
but somehow found strength, a will to repair.
For many men, toxic masculinity's cold embrace
Commands them sternly, leaving little space.
Man up, they're told. Don't shed a tear.
Be brave, unyielding. Show no hint of fear.
Don't be a girl, they hear from the early days.
Don't be gay, society's harsh phrase.
Such words like arrows pierce their tender hearts,
and leave them striving to play false parts.
Each day they fight to fit the rigid mould,
a tale of valour yet untold.
They shield those dear. Their shoulders bear the weight.
The price of strength, a burden they can't take.
Let's unshackle the chains that bind their souls
and embrace each heart, so they can feel whole.
Toxic expectations, let them fade —
As men and women let us lift the shade.
For only then in love's embrace
Shall burdened souls find peace and grace.

PULL YOUR SOCKS UP

Pull your socks up, they say with a grin.
Be a man. Hide the pain within.
But beneath this facade is our truth untold,
One sock up, one sock down, a soul in the cold.
I long for solace, a respite from strife.
Yet the pain persists, cutting like a knife.
Hope, they whisper – Hold On, Pain Ends.
But the pain lingers on, a foe that never bends.

I yearn for a way to escape this despair,
To find understanding, compassion, and care.
But the words keep echoing - be a man, stand tall,
as if emotions I must eternally forestall.
Pull your socks up, they say – they have no clue.
So let's redefine what it means to be true.
Seeking help is brave, don't harbour doubt
For sharing your burden – we'll figure it out.

MY TIME IS DONE

In January's grasp, my soul weighed down.
A burdened heart, a weary frown.
I made a list. Goodbyes to say.
Longing for the pain to end, the price to pay.
My struggles grew too much to bear,
Desperate whispers filled the air.
Today's the day my pain must cease.
A final act to find my peace.
To train tracks' edge my steps did wend,
With one resolve – my pain to end.

It needs to be swift, no turning back,
To avoid the burden of the survival track.
Convinced I was, I stole life's breath,
A weight upon my chest like death.
But as I stood on the rails' embrace,
Beyond the tracks, a different space.
Children played with laughter's glee,
Their innocence a sight to see.
They aimed their phones to film the train,
To capture joy and a moving game.
In their eyes they saw a man watching trains,
But in my heart a hidden truth, and pain.
Guilt. Shadows crept. My heart did pound.
How could they witness what I'd found?
A panic rose. I couldn't breathe.
A battle fought, as my broken soul sought
to find a way to break through the thought.
And even in my darkest hour,
Life's script held fast, with its timeless power.
I couldn't bear the weight of fate,
to seize control and meet Death's gate.
For deep inside a spark did stir,
A glimmer of hope, a voice that was sure.
Though darkness loomed, my heart did see
The children's smiles, the chance to be.
To hold on tight, to seek support,
To find my way, my last resort.
My time is done, I once believed,
But life is a journey not yet achieved.
In moments dark, seek out the light.
Embrace the day and hold on tight.

STAY ON THE RIGHT TRACK

Toxic masculinity and the media's glare.
It impacts women, a burden to bear.
Yet in the shadows, silently it creeps,
Affecting men three times more, there it sleeps.
As a society, we hold the key
To unlock the truth that all should see.
A responsibility we must embrace,
To show men a path towards a better place.
The most masculine thing they can do
Is take care of themselves. It's true.
Before attending to others' needs in plight,
Their superpower lies in self care's light.
Man up, they say. And so we find
The courage to face the trials behind.
For "man down" is a tragic call,
A loss for everyone, one and all.
Let's support boys from their early days,
To redefine what strength conveys.
Masculinity not defined by a frown,
But the heart as open, unafraid to drown.
It's okay not to be okay, we all proclaim.
Break the stigma, shatter the shame.
Generational bias we'll leave behind,
Leading from all sides a unified mind.
From top to bottom, and bottom to top.
Let's guide men, never let them drop.
Help them find the track that's right.
Celebrate their masculinity, shining bright.
For him, breaking barriers will unite
A world where hearts and souls ignite.
A place where boys can freely grow,
And men can face the highs and lows.

So let's stay on this path we've paved,
Where empathy and love are engraved;
Where strength is found in vulnerability,
And masculinity finds true nobility.

ONE IN TWENTY

One in 20. Whispers in the crowd,
Silent struggles, hearts wrapped in shroud.
Men – top banana they may seem,
Yet deep within they dare not to dream.
Thoughts of suicide. Shadows they chase.
Behind smiles, the darkness they embrace.
On the surface they wear a mask,
Inside their souls an ongoing task.
Just like bananas, slightly bruised
They're deemed imperfect, yet not abused.
For in the oven's warm embrace
Rotten bananas find their place.
In making bread they rise anew,
Transformed by care, as love seeps through.
It's never too late to find the way,
To bring them back from disarray.
Let's make banana bread together –
A stronger society bonded forever.
Masculine men unafraid to speak
Of struggles faced, emotions they seek.
Rotten bananas make great banana bread –
Likewise from pain, hope can be bred.
Together we'll rise, hearts intertwined.
One in 20 no longer confined.

Steve Whittle

CONTENTS

A BETTER HUMAN

Steve said my writing was a battle cry which inspired and empowered him, and now I've come to write this introduction, I'm sitting on a train crossing Canada from East to West wondering what to write and whether what comes next will do the men in this book, and around the world, justice.

Coming up with the idea of this book as I crossed the Atlantic Ocean, thinking of my two sons, I knew I wanted to collaborate with men on a book that helped everyone who read it become a better human.

Not just a better man, or a better woman.

A better human.

Surrounded by good men, very few were able, or willing, to step up for my sons following my divorce from their father, so I set out on the lonely journey of being a single mum raising boys.

My journey with men hasn't been an easy one, from being abandoned by my father, to discovering my ex-husband had been unfaithful throughout the eighteen years of our marriage, followed by narcissistic abuse from the partner who followed divorce, then violent sexual trauma. I could've very easily become a man hating, man bashing and emasculating woman, but that wasn't what I wanted.

I wanted to learn about men. I wanted a world where my boys were seen for the kind, caring protectors they are; celebrated for who they chose to be, and where the wounded women of the world didn't hurt them. I'd heard far too many hateful things come out of the mouths of women, and I knew that if women were ignored and abused the way these women were abusing men – to their faces and behind their backs – there would be massive public uproar.

With these two young men of mine, both very different in their physical attributes and ways of engaging with the world, preparing to embark on the world of work, I knew things were going to take a very different turn for them both. I wanted to prepare them for the world, but how could I when I myself didn't understand half the population?

Having read the stories you are about to read in this book, I've not only learned just how deeply men love, feel and grieve, but I've also discovered how they wish to provide and protect in ways I've never known or experienced.

Over my forty-six years, I've seen male youth workers, male teachers and men in general become the target of unfounded suspicions of being sexual predators. Men have been blamed for all problems in the world, and we've seen women encroach on male only spaces for fear of missing out, wanting to compete with men in every arena of life, and then blame men for the lack of success women face, when in many cases it is the moaning and victim mentality these women love to revel in that robs them of their success.

Since working on this book I've been called a men's rights activist, told I'm betraying women and that I'm self-serving, none of which are true. I may not be a man's rights activist but I am a human rights activist. I believe the more we understand others, the more we understand ourselves and the world we live in – and the closer we get to finding solutions for the many challenges we all face.

I'm deeply honoured that I've been gifted the trust of these men to bring their stories to life through this collaboration with Steve Whittle, the founder of Tough to Talk.

My hope is that this book will not only help raise awareness of the struggles and isolation men face, but also that it will help women to learn how to support the men in our lives, and how our actions and misguided beliefs are killing the men we love, destroying our communities and creating trauma that will last for many generations to come.

Some will have issues with the title #ManUp, but the antonym of man up is man down, and I for one, never want to see a man down, left behind or in pain. He is someone's son, and as a mother of sons, I am choosing to celebrate men, to lift them up, because what impacts man, impacts woman, both positively and negatively.

So here's to celebrating men in all their guises and helping them to #ManUp in the way they choose for themselves and overcome the challenges of the world together.

With love,

Founder of Dawn Publishing

MY WHY

BY STEVE WHITTLE

As an adult, I was diagnosed with complex PTSD (Post-Traumatic Stress Disorder), ADHD (Attention Deficit Hyperactivity Disorder), and depression, which I'd had for thirty-five years, and I wish I'd realised it and sought help sooner. It's fair to say I've always had mental health problems, but 2021 was a terrible year for me, culminating in my decision in early 2022 to take my own life for the third time.

In 2021, my life hit its peak. I have a great relationship, a fantastic job and a great circle of friends. Even so, every day, I felt like I was not contributing to those around me and regularly suffered from anxiety which sometimes manifested in panic attacks. This self-doubt cycle continued for months before hitting its peak in January 2022. I believed I was now not only *not* contributing to but *actually* detracting from the life of everyone around me.

My self-worth had turned into self-loathing, and I felt helpless. For months, I'd thought of completing suicide and had planned it out in my head. I'd thought of everything from my apology note to how to make it as final as possible. It was important not to survive the attempt and become an even more significant burden.

I suppose it didn't help that as a mental health first aider, I'd been signposting Dave, the chef, to help him with his mental health problems and keeping in regular contact with him. I was devastated to hear that he took his life whilst I was on holiday. I wondered whether, if I'd been around that week, we would have had enough contact for him to recognise his value to us all.

I sat in my home office thinking about all the people I would have to apologise to when I died. I opened up a Word document on my computer and started bullet-pointing the people to say sorry to. First, I put down the train driver, who had no idea I would ruin his day. Next, I put my girlfriend, mum, and son, and the list continued. After a while, I stopped putting reasons and just names. At that moment, I saw a list of people whose lives I had made worse by being in it. I had let them all down and had not fulfilled my potential. They would all be better off without me.

I set my computer not to shut down and left the apology note on the screen. I left the house and walked to the train crossing about ten minutes away. There was one next to my house, but it was always busy, and I wanted to avoid the fuss of anyone seeing me. I stood leaning on the gate that leads to the train tracks waiting for the next train and going over in my head what I would do to make sure this worked.

It was all about timing: don't come out too soon so the driver brakes or too late to avoid getting under the train. This needs to be final.

Some children started playing on the opposite side of the tracks, about ten metres away. They were laughing and joking. They saw me and made eye contact but continued enjoying themselves. The train was coming, and I got myself ready. I was confident this was the right thing to do and planned to step out when the train reached a certain point on the tracks.

The children saw the train coming too and climbed up on the gate opposite to watch it pass, and one got their mobile phone out to video it. As the train approached, I started to think about how this would affect them, watching me throw myself under the train in front of them. The train reached my stepping-out point, and I looked at the kids... and I didn't step out, and I'm not sure why I hesitated.

I missed my opportunity but knew I'd be ok. There would be another train shortly, and the children would hopefully be gone. Eventually, I was alone again, waiting for the next train. I was still thinking about how this would have affected the children and how a video of my suicide would impact my girlfriend and family. I started to feel guilty, but this only added to why everyone was better off without me. I began to think about Big Dave and what it must have been like for his family to find out how he took his life and if they knew why he felt so undervalued.

Feeling out of control and sick, I started with a panic attack and tried to control it. I began to walk it off and control my breathing. When I felt some control, I was back home and in my office, staring at the apology list. I felt humiliated and a failure. Look at me back home; I can't even manage to kill myself. This feeling worsened because this wasn't the first time I had failed.

A while passed, and I had a moment of clarity. I was unsure what made me ask for help, but I contacted the NHS support line and told them what happened. They were sympathetic without being patronising. The therapist knew what to say and asked many questions to ensure I wasn't in immediate danger.

They talked to me for a long time and would only hang up once they were convinced I would be ok until they could get me support. I was given some advice to let those closest to me know what I was going through so they could support me. I agreed but knew there was no way I was doing that. I felt humiliated that I had let myself get in such a bad way and had to get help. The last thing I needed was for those around me to see how weak and pathetic I was. I can do this independently with the help of strangers without burdening those closest to me.

The NHS (National Health Service) gave me emergency counselling but had assessed that I needed trauma counselling, which would take up to six months. After a few sessions, the counsellor said she was discharging me, and I was to wait for the trauma sessions. There were not enough councillors for the number of people needing urgent help.

I hit a new low in February as my work started to suffer. My boss had picked up on this, and rightly so. She arranged a meeting with me to chat. I interpreted that as 'I'm getting fired; I've failed again' and prepared for the worst. I tried to pre-empt the conversion in the meeting and head her off by recognising my work failures and explaining that I could turn them around.

She let me burn myself out and waited for me to stop talking. She told me she didn't care about the work. She wanted me to know she had noticed a significant change in my behaviour. My outlook and attitude had changed, and people were worried about me. Of course, I reacted defensively to this and tried to play it down. Brilliantly, she let me talk myself out again and waited for me to finish.

She reassured me that everything was ok and I shouldn't worry about work. She explained that she was worried about me and that I was her primary concern, that my welfare was vital to her and the company. She said it was ok not to talk to her about what was happening to me, but if I did, she wouldn't judge me and would listen. I'm not sure how I told her what was going on. My memory is a blur. I think I just rattled out all my problems, including the suicide attempt, like a machine gun.

I had never felt so vulnerable and was sure she would brush me off or laugh at me and tell me to pull my socks up. We had a great conversation, and she showed incredible empathy and helped me develop a plan for the next steps. I agreed to speak to my girlfriend that night about my feelings and suicide attempt, take some leave and book in with the GP immediately. She asked me if she could share what I was going through with HR to see what support work could offer me. I agreed but was worried. This was the turning point for me, finally finding the strength to talk it through and the persistence of someone willing to listen and not judge.

> IMPORTANT SIDE NOTE: Of course, those closest to me, like my girlfriend, would have reacted exactly as Mel did, but I would never have willingly opened up to them, as I have always seen myself as their protector. It's a man thing, and this is the stigma we need to work together to destroy.

My GP and I agreed to start medication and wait for the trauma counselling. Through work, I started trauma coaching through Sanctus. I was dubious about sharing my issues with a stranger, but it was life-changing... and terrifying. I also had three months off work to get my shit together.

So how am I now? Well, I'm in a much better place and have a structure to help manage my mental health. Seriously, I have a healthy relationship with myself and those around me and a passion not to become so unwell again.

I do have days when I'm not "top banana", and I know the best thing to do is tell those closest to me, use the protocols I've learned through coaching and trust the process. I've made that sound easy, but it's not - it's still tough to talk about things when I'm having a bad day. It isn't easy for anyone to suffer, and I hope you speak, like I eventually did, if you are struggling.

I've shared my story to let people know it can happen to anyone and show you all that without the help of those around me, I wouldn't be here to tell that story. I would love to inspire those who need help to seek it and those who might be worried about someone to help in any way they can.

My personal experience and the pivotal conversation with my boss served as catalysts for establishing the charity Tough to Talk. The willingness of individuals to Break The Silence, engage in challenging dialogues, and show vulnerability fuelled the formation of this charity. I'm not referring to those enduring pain but to those courageous souls who act upon what they see, hear and know about others' struggles. They muster the strength and courage to raise their voices, assisting those who may feel helpless and hopeless. By Breaking The Silence, destroying the stigma, and intervening to support men in need, we endeavour to save lives, one at a time.

ONE

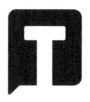

GRIEF: ADAM

Being fifty-six years old means I was born in the mid-1960s, which I believe is relevant because attitudes were vastly different then about what is a man and how a man should behave. I had a happy childhood despite my parents divorcing when I was three or four. My mum and my nan brought me up and they did a rather decent job of it. I was happy at school; I'm quite academic and I'm told I'm quite intelligent.

My mum remarried, and I got on really well with my stepdad and my stepbrother and stepsister. When I was thirteen, nearly fourteen, my mum suddenly passed away, which is quite clearly a big deal, and I think I had some unresolved issues because of that for many years.

My stepdad remarried a woman who never had children, which meant she didn't understand teenagers, especially not a fifteen-year-old teenager like I was at the time. This resulted in several arguments, culminating in me being thrown out six weeks before my O-Levels. So I ended up living in a one-bedroom flat with my grandmother, sleeping on a camp bed that had been donated by one of her cousins. That was incredibly difficult, but my grandmother was a wonderful woman, and I was the apple of her eye, which made everything lovely.

As a single parent, my mum had worked two jobs. She was a bookkeeper by day and a photographer in the evenings and at weekends, so my grandmother raised me; and then she had to bury her daughter, which no parent ever imagines having to do – that's not the way the world is supposed to work. And suddenly at age seventy-something, she had a teenager in her home that she was responsible for.

When I was twenty-three, my grandmother passed away, so I was now on my own, as by this time I had no contact with my stepdad or my stepbrother and stepsister. I just had to get on with things.

The twenty-three-year-old me was vastly different to fourteen-year-old me, and even though it was a massive loss to lose my grandmother, who had effectively brought me up, she'd been with me longer than my mum had. The grief was different.

At twenty-three, when she died, I understood better. She had a stroke, went into hospital and was clinging on for the best part of three months. I firmly believe that she clung on because she felt that she needed to look after me still. She was unconscious most of the time towards the end, and eventually I just said to her, 'It's okay, I'll be fine. You can rest now.' And she passed that night.

I think the significant difference, other than the fact that I was nine years older, is that I was prepared. I knew it was the right thing. Whereas with my mum, I went to school that morning and she kissed me at the door, said she loved me, and the next thing I knew, I was told I needed to go home. Even though I was prepared for the death of my grandmother, the way I dealt with it was to bury my feelings.

In regard to my career, you could say I fell into information technology, something I really enjoyed. In the mid-eighties I started working my way up the career ladder, until 2016 when I became IT director of a now well-known construction company, which was brilliant – that was my dream job. I felt like I'd arrived. I'd achieved my primary ambition from a career perspective, and I was incredibly happy, doing well salary-wise, and so on.

During my career climb I met my wife, and in 1995 we got married. We had our two sons in 1997 and 1999. And then things started to go wrong, and I realised my wife was quite abusive. She had an interesting relationship with her mum where they saw each other every day. And then, when they weren't together, they'd be on the phone. When we moved from Southeast London to East Kent, a week later her mum and dad moved from Southeast London to East Kent. They were always very, very close to each other.

My ex-wife came from a family that were proper Southeast Londoners – her grandad was one of the original members of the SAS in World War 2, the Dirty Dozen, when they recruited people from military prison. After the war, he stayed behind in Germany for two years because he had a German girlfriend, and when he came back he was a boxer and once fought someone who went on to become world champion. But he was a product of his environment, and he was quite abusive to his wife, and this abuse filtered down through the generations.

My wife was absolutely infatuated with the idea of having a daughter of her own so that she could have a similar relationship to the one she had with her own mother; but we had to have fertility treatment because she had polycystic ovaries, and we were blessed with two sons.

When the twenty-week scan showed we were having a second boy, the relationship with my wife took an absolute nosedive as she blamed me for not giving her a daughter. The change in her was like flicking a switch. It started off as verbal abuse – 'It's your fault, you're responsible for the sex of the baby, you know how much I wanted a daughter, why can't you give me a daughter?' I knew it was irrational, but it was constant, and I learned to just put up with it. It then became physical, and again I put up with it, because as a child of the sixties, you never raise your hand to a woman, you just learn to soak it up, so that's what I did.

I think I stayed there because, being the product of a broken home, I felt it was important that my children didn't have the issues that go along with having your family broken. However, things got worse and worse, and ultimately that drove me to have an affair. It's not like I woke up one morning and thought, 'Right, I'm going to go and find myself someone else.' That's absolutely not what happened.

A lot of people saw my affair as the cause of the marriage breakup, including my boys initially, because they were too young at the time for me to be able to tell them that their mother was abusive to me. Even when I did tell them, only relatively recently, I debated long and hard because I didn't want to taint their memory of their mum. My wife and I eventually got divorced in 2012, and the boys were shocked but not surprised. It would have been obvious to anybody that things weren't going well, but it still comes as a shock to you when your parents sit you down and say, guys, we're separating.

When she passed away from what is called a carcinoid, a neuroendocrine cancer, things became quite difficult because I didn't really know how to feel. I'd looked after my boys, and the Child Support Agency (CSA) weren't required, as I'd paid way over the odds in maintenance and kept them in the home they were all used to, which I admit I resented. I didn't have to do that, but it became the expectation, and I personally felt it was the right thing to do. Again, being a man born in the 1960s, you provide for your family, you're strong and everything is fine. You keep your head high and you carry on. Today it is different, and so I struggled to relate to my boys. The construction company I was working for could see I was struggling and funded me seeing a counsellor, as I had genuine issues at this time. The company was very good in that respect. I don't know whether the counsellor was good, bad, or average, but I think it helped. It felt to me like I was sitting and speaking, and what I was getting back wasn't what I felt was practical advice. It was an opportunity for forty-five minutes to purge and vent, which helped to an extent. I didn't get any real practical strategies or coping mechanisms, and I would have liked some real insight into the psychology behind what I was going through, to help me understand what was going on in my brain. Some strategies to help me sleep, to help me cope, to help me know what to do about the rage, the sadness, the hopelessness would have been ideal, but I got what I got.

I can't say that I ever experienced any stigma or discrimination to do with the difficulties I had, as society had started to understand it for what it is and not see my struggles as a sign of weakness. Had this happened in my teenage years – which obviously it didn't, because I kept it all bottled up – if I'd been seeing a counsellor, it might have been different; kids are cruel.

Although I don't know what it would be like now, in 2023, I'd like to think that kids are a little bit kinder. Then you read about the likes of Caroline Flack and others who on the surface seem to have got it all, but have taken their own lives, and you do wonder how it would have turned out if people had been kinder.

Would people have been kinder to someone like Phillip Schofield if it had been a female colleague that he'd had a relationship with? You see #bekind trending, but then you see something that makes you think, hang on a minute, you might not like what someone's done, or is doing, but if it's legal and consensual, then butt out ... and be kind.

Both my boys have recently gone through their teenage years, which I had to deal with alone. They don't live with me, and they've obviously suffered a devastating loss – and that's been quite difficult for me, bearing in mind my residual feelings about their mum, which I obviously can't voice to them yet. But I felt I needed to be a sponge and take on their grief, their regret, their resentment. They have unresolved issues and won't speak with counsellors, as has been suggested. It's difficult for me as I'm not trained to have the kind of conversations with my boys they need to have, nor am I trained to hear the kinds of things to then be able to put them aside.

Of course, they're my children, so as a parent we can't just compartmentalise the grief and divorce. The other difficulty is that because she was the one they lost, and I'm the one left behind, she's been kind of canonised, while I've been demonised, and that makes for a difficult relationship, particularly with my younger son.

Looking back, I realise that when my mum passed away, I didn't get angry, and I don't really remember crying much. My stepdad was very much "You need to be strong and keep your chin up." This was 1980, and nowadays more services are available to kids of that age to give them the opportunity to talk about it.

That was not available to me, and so I think I just bottled it up. My memory of it is kind of hazy if I'm honest, and I wish we could have had this conversation forty years ago. When you're fourteen, your peers don't take you aside and say, "How are you feeling?", "How are things?", "Is everything okay?", "Is there anything I can do?" That's just not what teenagers do – well, it wasn't then, I don't know about now.

The financial implications of sorting out my ex-wife's estate were difficult. The boys got a lot of the money, which they've not done anything useful with whatsoever. This is something else I feel resentful about because I worked a long, long time, and very hard, to get to a position where I could provide them with the kind of environment, security, and inheritance they have received.

Despite all the issues in my family life, I was in love with my job, in love with the business. The company I worked for was Rydon Construction, the lead developer on the refurbishment of Grenfell Tower. The Grenfell Tower works happened before I even joined the company, but clearly that hit the business extremely hard, which resulted in my role being made redundant in 2018. I know people say, "I was made redundant", but I think it's right to say my *role* was made redundant – I'd done a really good job, but they were able to survive without me, and they had to think about the fact that my salary was well into six figures, plus a director's bonus.

The redundancy hit me hard. I wouldn't be able to rank where all these life events are set in terms of the one that's hit me hardest, but there's definitely been a cumulative effect and the impact has been quite huge.

Simultaneously, my then-partner's role in financial services was also made redundant and we went from being a quarter-of-a-million-pounds-a-year couple to zero income. The impact on our life was harsh. We'd been renting in Surrey due to my work, and my partner had sold her house in South Wales so we could move in together. So we found ourselves in our fifties with no property, no assets, and we found ourselves wondering what we were going to do.

We chose to move to Derbyshire, and I love Derbyshire, love Derby, love the people, love everything about it. My partner and I had been discussing the seed of an idea about setting up a photography business since 2018. We'd thought about opening a café, and thank God we didn't, as COVID would have added that to the catalogue of disasters!

We went ahead with the photography, and our work is considered by our peers to be exceedingly high quality, although at the start there's an element of faking it until you make it and having that bravado blend well with focus and determination to succeed.

It's still difficult for me to talk about my feelings, even though I know it's not showing weakness; that's what it feels like. For example, I've got somewhere around two thousand connections on LinkedIn who know me as a strong, no-nonsense IT director. My teams, the people that work for me, the young people that I've nurtured, trained, and mentored, they know me as someone who's strong, who gets things done, who's fair, caring, all those things. And so it's difficult for me even to go on LinkedIn and say, "Actually, I'm really struggling." Because that's not the persona that I've carefully created over fifty years.

The way you feel hits you in different ways. It can come at you from nowhere, and the smallest thing can cause you rage, or sadness, or hopelessness. But I deal with it ... because that's what men do.

All these things come back to being a child of the sixties – this is the man's role, you're a provider, you're the pillar of strength for the family, you don't show weakness, you don't cry. And you certainly don't let other people know that you're struggling.

And that's wrong.

Obviously, I'm not a trained professional, but I think that's the essence of toxic masculinity – whatever you're going through, don't show it, keep the mask on.

There were good things about the old ways of being a man: I always walk kerb side when I'm out with my partner, so in case a carriage comes by and splashes us, I take the splash. I hold doors open. I won't sit down until she's sat down. So it's not all bad.

We need to get past this whole thing of "I can't show that I'm struggling."

I would say that my strength now, in today's version of myself, is that I'm still here – a lot of people wouldn't be.

My superpower now is to be able to say to people, no matter how shit it gets, no matter what happens to you, it's not the end, there is a light at the end of the tunnel, and it is perfectly possible to be a functioning member of society, despite all the hardships that you've had.

Everybody goes through these things – at some point in your life you will lose your grandparents, you will lose your parents, you'll lose a job. We adapt and survive. I'm pragmatic now, but sometimes there is that thing in the back of my head that sort of drags me back to the toxic masculinity way of being.

There are some things that I worry about now that I don't articulate to my partner because I don't want to worry her. There's absolutely no danger that I'm going to "check myself out." I have considered it over the years, but that's not my thing – I feel it's an unnecessary solution to a problem.

There is help available, but you must access it, it won't come looking for you.

As I've got older, I've started to believe in the power of karma. I wouldn't say I was a spiritual person, but I I'd like to think that if I give, then eventually good things will start happening.

For anyone going through struggles similar to mine, my advice would be talk to someone.

I'd tell my fourteen-year-old self to talk to a teacher, because they have access to the kind of services you need. I didn't do that, and I had unresolved issues for many years, I was angry. I've told my boys that they need to get some counselling, to talk to someone, and it's important to have those conversations when things are fine. *Not when you're losing your shit, and you're irrational, and you're arguing with your partner.*

Talk to the counsellor when you're lucid and articulate and can absorb the information they're giving you, then you'll have those coping mechanisms to use when you need them.

REFLECTIONS

REFLECTIONS

REFLECTIONS

TWO

ISOLATION: ROB

My entire childhood was tough. I was early in development when it came to reading, writing and calculating, which became a bit of a problem for me the entire time I was at school.

In Sweden you have preschool for one year before you start first grade. It's not mandatory, you don't need to go, at least not when I was young. As my birthday is in December, I was five years old turning six when I started school, and my sister was already in school. She started learning English when she was in third grade, but before that I stole her books to learn how to read and write and develop the other skills she was learning.

My dad was very supportive, and my mum also helped me to get a little bit ahead of everyone, encouraging me to learn new stuff and be curious about everything.

When I started first grade, I had a different dialect from everyone else in the school because when I was born, we moved to from Gävle to Skåne, in the southern part of Sweden. I started learning to talk when I was living there, and then we moved to Borlänge, which is in the centre of Sweden. By that point, I had this strange dialect which no one could understand. Also, when I started first grade I was already at third grade level in Swedish language, calculating and additional subjects; add to that the fact that I started learning English the year before my peers did.

This became a big problem for me for my entire time in school. When I started high school things were a little bit better, although my sister had already taken high school classes, which meant I was continually borrowing her books and started high school mathematics, chemistry and physics earlier than most, putting me even further ahead of my classmates.

In ninth grade, aged fifteen, I did some school projects. I had to go beyond the schoolbooks because I was bored in school, so I borrowed some books from the Royal Institute of Technology in Sweden. I started reading about nanotechnology, which was a very new concept in the early 1990s. I got bullied for my entire life because I was so much smarter than others.

We have something here in Sweden, more of an unwritten rule, that you should never brag. You're not better than anyone. You're just mediocre, and that is shown in everything we do here in Sweden.

For example, all men have the same dark clothes. There are no colours here. Everyone is going about their business in the same way. No one stands out, because if you stand out from the crowd, then you're going to get attention, and we shouldn't get any attention.

It's a bit of a problem because when you have a story you shouldn't make it a big deal; you shouldn't talk about yourself, that's not a good way to do. That's the way we have been brought up for a very long time here in Sweden, but it tends to be shifting right now for the millennials. I'm the generation that went on a bike without a helmet. We climbed trees to the third floor, and no one cared. You fall, you break a leg, shit happens; so I am quite resilient in many ways, as many adults my age are.

In 1993 I was eighteen, and I met a girl whom I later got engaged to, and we eventually moved in together. At first, the relationship was good. It was my first real relationship, so I didn't have anything to compare it to. Before we moved in together, I asked my girlfriend if she was coming over and she said, "No, I'm kind of busy", and I said, "Yeah, OK, no problem, no problem." I didn't think anything of it. In 1996, we moved in together, and then in 1997 we broke up and she moved out, because it turns out that she was cheating on me for four years with my best friend. And that was the point my entire life started to go down the drain.

Later in 1997, I met a new girlfriend. We were together for a year and then I discovered she was also cheating on me, which further degraded my problems. I met a new girl several years later in 2001. We broke up in 2003 because she met a new guy at a school trip, and so after that I've been alone more or less.

This kind of betrayal has broken me in so many ways that I have trust issues. I cannot trust anyone, and it has given me a lot of social problems. The betrayals are the main reason why I lost my footing.

In 2006 I was friends with new people. We had parties and got together; I had a "friend with benefits" but for some reason I got more depressed. She told me, "You need to go to see someone." I took her advice and went to a psychiatrist. Her approach was like the teachings of Freud, in terms that it was like, "OK, so what's your problem? Why do you need help? What? Why?" It was horrible. I went to see another doctor and he gave me medications which didn't work.

I still didn't feel so good, so we did this survey that rates how you are in terms of self-harm, suicide prevention, and depression.. I filled out that form and it showed that I was having a high probability of suicide.

The doctor said, "You know what? This is very high. You've been on medication for several months. I don't like this. You have two options. Either you go to the hospital, and you get hospitalised for as long as we deem necessary, or you go through the ECT programme." I opted for the ECT (electroconvulsive therapy) programme and had ECT six times. This helped in the sense that for several years I didn't have any thoughts of killing or harming myself.

Electroconvulsive therapy, which was shown in the movie *One Flew Over the Cuckoo's Nest*, works by jump-starting your brain with electricity.

Unlike in the movie, here in Sweden they give you a sedative and muscle relaxant so you don't bite your tongue or feel the pain. What they're fundamentally doing is inducing an epileptic attack to restart the brain. The downside is that you might lose short-term memory, which I've experienced. My memory is better now than it was, but it was tough for a while, forgetting where I put my phone when it was in my hand.

Everything was good for a couple of years, even when I started university, because I started university at thirty-four. My situation got worse whilst I was at university, especially in the last year. I counted that I'd had depression for at least fifteen years, give or take, with the latest incident being a few months ago.

I was with some people whom I'd considered friends, but it turned out they only wanted information from me, as I was working for Swedish Immigration and had a lot of knowledge about permits and coming to Sweden. They told me to my face, "No, we're not friends. I just needed information." And I thought, 'Hmm, OK'. We'd gone for fika, which is a very big part of Swedish culture and consists of having coffee, tea or a soft drink together with some pastries. But it's more than that. It's like when you go to a football game, you don't go there just to watch twenty-two guys kick a ball, you go there for the mood, the everything around it. It's an entire experience. My mind kept thinking, 'How is this possible?' It didn't make sense to me. So when I left, I went by the water to get to the subway, and thought, 'Maybe I should try to swim to Finland', which is not going to happen when it's -10 outside and the water is freezing. I wouldn't get very far, but that was the entire point of it. It was a really bad moment for me.

After that I talked to a colleague, and she forced me to get in touch with someone. Which meant that I had to have an appointment with the emergency psychology team in Stockholm. I went, had some conversations, and now I'm seeing a therapist. I'm not sure what it's going to give me because I don't respond to medications. I haven't slept properly since 2006.

Deep down inside me, there is something that stops me from

taking the plunge, so to speak. I don't know what it is, but it's something, because it's not the first time I've thought about suicide. I can honestly say that for the last few months it's been a reoccurring thought in my head that maybe I should do something.

Here in Stockholm, it's quite popular to throw yourself in front of a train or jump from high bridges. For me, the thought of a train is it's quick, it's painless, but there's someone driving the train. I don't want to scar anyone else. So in some way I stop myself from doing anything because that thought is still nagging me all the time.

The therapy I'm in now is behavioural activation therapy, which means to be active, to meet people, to do stuff. For me, I tried to do that. I know a lot of people; I'm not friends with them, but I know a lot of people so I'm trying to figure out things to do. Meeting new people here in Stockholm is difficult. The Swedish culture is a very closed culture where to be part of a group means that you need to have an entry point to that group. If you don't have any friends, it's difficult to get new friends. Swedes are very closed people until you get to know them, and when you do, they open up a lot.

That is the main problem for me, and that is also one thing that my therapist and I are trying to focus on. However, the advice I get for the moment is to try to find a group that has an interest similar to mine, but that's crazy expensive. To do courses and stuff like that, it's really expensive. On a government salary here in Sweden, you *cannot* rent an apartment in Stockholm. I don't work in Stockholm, I work in Uppsala, which is an hour and a half by train, so I commute three hours per day. Some days I work from home, which is nice, but otherwise the time is a big problem, and the salary is not that good, which means I cannot afford to go to these clubs or do these activities.

There is a stigma and discrimination here in Sweden, and I can say that not many in my proximity know about my problems. Neither my mum nor sister knows anything about my problems, and they're the only family I have left. My dad passed away in 2005. Not all my family knows. I have one friend and she knows everything, but we don't have that much connection or contact anymore. Most people will say, "Just go out, go have fun", and the other common thing is "man up". We use a different term here in Sweden, but it all boils down to "man up".

Discrimination doesn't happen as no one knows about it. There are three bosses I've talked to about my problems over the years, so they understand if I need to go from work early, leave in the middle of the day, or just be at home, and they know there might be problems. My first boss offered fake sympathy. He is borderline psychopath and everyone at that unit had the same problem. Real feelings are not his thing.

However, the team supervisors, they were very supportive. I needed to move to a different unit, the one in Uppsala, and my boss there was very understanding. He didn't react the way I thought he would.

My first boss had asked, "What am I going to do about it? Deal with it." That was the fear I had, and then my next boss told me, "If there's anything I can do, just tell me. If you need time off, tell me. If you need to go to see someone, tell me. Do whatever you want. Just tell me. No problem." It was good, really uplifting, because then I knew that it didn't matter and that I had the support.

The Saturday night I mentioned before about the person who I thought was a friend and who told me he was only using me for information, the night when my emotions crashed and I was planning to take the swim to Finland – I texted my boss early on Monday morning and said, "I'm not coming to work, I crashed this weekend", and he replied directly in a few minutes and said, "Take your time. No problem." It was nice to know that I didn't have to go to work and feel like a big piece of crap.

I've learnt to talk to someone as soon as possible, especially if I'm feeling suicidal, and I recommend talking with people about what is going on.

I believe it would've helped me when I was a kid, but no one knew exactly what was wrong with me. Of course, they thought I had ADHD, so they did something called WISC, an intelligence test to see if you have any problems like ADHD. It turns out that I didn't answer the easy questions. I only answered the hard questions. No one cared which was important in 2009. When I had a friend that said, "I'm going to take the test for Mensa, and I want you to come with me", I replied, "Why should I do that? I'm not going to be a part of that organisation, so why should I?" He nagged at me, and then it turned out he didn't have a car, so he couldn't go to the test because it was a very long drive. In the end, I signed up for the test in May 2009, so I drove us there. I received my letter from Mensa when they'd tallied all the results, and I got the answer to why I am the way I am. They cannot measure my IQ; it's off the scale and I'm in the top 1%.

I usually say that I got lucky on the test, because sometimes I feel really stupid, but this result also makes a whole lot of sense since it kind of hinders my social development, which I've a hard time with, even now. I can't talk to people in difficult situations. I know how to have an investigation, interrogation, everything like that, but that's about it; I don't have any social skills. I know that in some ways I am better than a lot of people, and in some ways I really suck at things. I'm great at logic, but social skills, not so much.

Due to my experiences and struggles, I've a hard time trusting people, which has shaped my personal growth and resilience. People ask me to go for fika, and at work it is mandatory to have these breaks. If you don't take a break, the boss will say, "You need to take a break" or ask, "Do you need to go to have a fika?"

When I get asked to go for fika, I automatically come to the conclusion that we're not going to meet up, we're not going to do anything, nothing is going to happen. If I make plans with someone, I ask someone, "Should we go out just to have a drink" or something, they say, "Yeah, of course." Then I automatically think, the same day we're going to go out, that they're going to call me or text me. And then they text me, "Oh, I cannot come", "Oh no, I need to work", "I'm too tired" or "I'm sick" and it disappoints me every time, all the time in fact, so I'm afraid to make plans. I'm afraid to keep my hopes up, to put myself out there, because I know I'm going to get hurt again.

I was at the point where I found the opportunity to be vulnerable, even though it was by accident, and my friend received it so well. My fear was that if I show any kind of vulnerability it will be received negatively, because we're supposed to be strong and stoic. This has been my fear for my entire life because when I was bullied as a kid, that was when I started to get this "stone face" that nothing bothered me. I didn't show anyone, not even my parents. I've been acting for at least around forty years.

It all comes back to talking to somebody as soon as you notice the signs that you are not OK, because when I had my first breakdown in 2007 and I had the ECT, I was ignoring all the signs. I ignored everything. And before this time, when I broke down, when my friend told me, "You need to go see someone", I'd say, "yeah, yeah, I will." I was trying to avoid it, until she took me into her room and said, "Now, you're going to call someone and you're going to need to call them tonight. Not whenever. Call them tonight. When you've done that, you text me. You text me right away. If you do not do that, I will come and hunt you tomorrow. And I will make sure that you call them tomorrow." I thought she was super annoying, and I told her, "No, just leave me alone, go away." But then I started thinking that yeah, she's right. I started looking at myself and saw all these signs that I'd had such a long time ago, which led me to the most invasive procedure you can have in psychology: putting someone to sleep just to fry their brain with electricity. I said to myself, "No freaking way I'm going to go through that again. That isn't going to happen!" before telling myself, "She's right. I'm going to do this."

I'm grateful to this friend because she was the one who noticed that I wasn't feeling very good. I'd never told her directly and I don't remember exactly what we were talking about. But she saw through my normal "stone face" when I'm talking with people. I'm an expert at hiding my feelings, and I should get an Oscar for my performance. But she said something that made my face crack a little bit, and she saw that a tear was forming in my eye. And that's when she reacted immediately. And I was "Oh crap! This is not good", but it turned out that she was very supportive, and she still is.

Regarding prioritising and managing my mental health long term, I have no clue at all what to do. These livestreams that Tough to Talk put on I've found quite helpful in the sense that I get some kind of therapy, because I see all the comments that people make and how they talk about their different stories. That makes me feel like I'm not alone in this, which feels good. Even though it doesn't help the problem or solve my issues, it's still a little bit on the way to healing myself.

REFLECTIONS

REFLECTIONS

REFLECTIONS

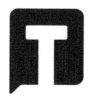

THREE

ABUSE: CARL

I'm going to go right back to the beginning of my story: I was sexually abused by my uncle, on my mother's side, when I was five. It happened once to me, and also to my sister, which is when my dad caught him and went ape s**t.

The uncle who did this is behind on his mental development, so he seemed five or ten years younger than he actually was. How are you supposed to deal with that? It made me question a lot when I was younger, my sexuality and all sorts, but I don't think it really affected me until a couple of years ago.

When I was around six years old, I came home from school one day and caught my mother cheating with my dad's brother. A couple of days later I was out fishing with my dad – we were pretty avid fishermen – and I mentioned it, just innocently; it was just something I'd seen. He went home and had an argument with them. They denied the affair and I was called a liar. I was made to apologise to my uncle, and my dad gave me a good clout for lying. After three or four weeks, my mum and uncle admitted to having an affair, and everything broke down for me. I was blamed for it all by both my parents, and up to this day they've never admitted they were wrong or that I was telling them the truth.

My dad made me choose between him and my mum when they split up, and having seen what I'd seen, I chose my dad. Then my dad started going out with other women, and I was overlooked because the women were all my dad was interested in.

I then went to live with my mum, at which point she'd remarried, and my stepfather started physically abusing me. Every chance he got, he'd punch me in the face or headbutt me. I think it was a way for him to get his anger out. He's still with my mum now, thirty-odd years later.

Never being able to fully express myself as a child resulted in a lot of anger issues because my feelings weren't expressed. I think if you can't express yourself, you're never going to really find a good path in life. I never physically abused other people; my anger was always directed at smashing things.

In my mid to late teens, I was addicted to amphetamine for about two years and had a pretty bad addiction at one point. I can't even reflect on back then, to be honest; all I know is that I was addicted to this drug and this drug was all I cared about.

I worked eighteen hours for four days at a time, then went out drinking on the days I was off and just took the drug. That was my life for about two years. I also became addicted to cannabis for around twelve years, and I've only recently come off that, because of the paranoia it was causing me.

From the time I was eighteen to age thirty-five, I'd say I had regular breakdowns. The only way I can explain what I was experiencing is that it's kind of like a balloon: when you put air into the balloon and it gets to a point where it just explodes because there's nowhere for the air to escape to. That's what it's like. That overwhelming feeling, like a burning sensation in the pit of your stomach, and you start to question why you're around people, why people are around you. An example is when my wife says to me that she loves me, and I say, "No, you don't," because I can't believe that I'm of benefit to people.

Why do people really want me around in their lives? I've no idea. The anxieties these feelings create are difficult to describe. The closest thing I can think of is, it's a bit like if you're sitting between two people and every minute those people move closer and closer to you until they're literally on your lap. You start to feel hemmed in, and then it's like an explosion of pure anger. After the anger, it's just emotion, crying my eyes out and breaking down. I've never taken medication for depression or anything like that because I'm so emotionally aware. I just deal with it, managing the symptoms by trying to understand them. I ask myself why I'm so angry, why I'm snapping at people, then I'll start to develop hatred towards myself, which is when I start punching stuff and wanting to see blood from my fists. I've got scars all over my hands.

I went through a breakup with my ex when I was in my early twenties, and I had to fight social services to get custody of our daughter. My ex was addicted to drugs for many years, and she was neglecting our daughter. I remember getting a phone call when she was two or three years old from a friend, saying she'd turned up at their house at 3:00 am. When I went to pick her up, I discovered that her mother had passed out on the sofa at home after taking heroin, leaving our daughter playing in dog s**t in the kitchen before walking over to the friend's house. My daughter has been through a period of self-harm as a result of her early childhood. She started cutting herself when she was a teenager – fortunately, she doesn't do it anymore.

My violent outbursts mean I don't have any friends. I had friends before, but they saw me being 90 per cent okay, happy-go-lucky and helping people, and then they'd see the 10 per cent that they didn't like, and they'd tend to walk away from that. My anger makes people question the person they think they know, and they don't stay in my life long enough for me to explain and help them to understand.

I was always an active person, always on the go, fast-paced, working sixty–seventy hours a week, kickboxing, going to the gym. But around two years ago I developed Crohn's disease and I've had to slow everything down. My exercise went down to zero, and I work part time.

Those who have Crohn's disease experience it differently from one another, and for me it's moderate discomfort, but all the time, with occasional flare-ups. I was also caring for my current wife, who has her own mental health issues (she suffers from paranoid schizophrenia), and I just didn't know where to turn. Being a man, there's an expectation that comes with that. When you try to talk to people, their reaction is that you've been this strong guy all this time, and now all of a sudden you're showing weakness.

All these different aspects of my trauma, the bullying, physical abuse, mental abuse, rejection, everything, started to surface shortly after I was diagnosed. All these bad memories started to creep up. It was so overwhelming that I ended up losing the plot.

Looking back from where I am now, I can see the patterns. I can see these violent outbursts I have, and the drug addiction was how I managed the outbursts, how I dealt with things. I've had to dissect a lot of stuff since I got Crohn's disease, stuff that should've been fixed at the time and is now an overwhelming thing that's constantly hovering over me.

I get lots of different emotions that all come at me within minutes of each other, and it's hard to regulate that sort of thing. As I wasn't able to express myself as a child, I find it difficult now to express myself because I wasn't taught the skills for self-expression. I was pushed away for telling the truth to my father, so I wouldn't tell people what I felt because I was worried about how they'd react.

The problem with trying to get help, for me at the moment, is that I've got such a vast array of trauma that I've got to reach out to five or six different charities to find people to help me deal with each one individually.

In 2015, I attempted suicide. I'd recently lost my grandfather, who I relied on for support and guidance, and I didn't have anyone else left to support me. I was also dealing with my wife's mental health issues, all of this on my own. Part of my wife's condition is that she has major anger issues and can say some really hateful things. She wasn't getting the help she needed, and I was the only support and help she had. She has been violent towards me in the past, but I've invited it because I'd rather she hurt me than hurt herself.

In 2015 we had a big bust-up and I was at a very low point. She told me she hated me and it was over. I drove off in the car up onto the mountain nearby, and I parked on the edge of a cliff. I was revving the engine, ready to pop off and just go for it.

Then my daughter called me.

It was very unusual for my daughter to call me, so I presumed my wife must have spoken to her. She told me my wife had tried calling me and I wasn't answering, so she called me. Speaking with my daughter changed my mind about my suicide attempt. She asked me what I was doing, and as soon as I heard her voice everything just went down a couple of levels. I didn't tell her at the time where I was or what I was planning.

Being in the car, looking over the edge of the cliff, I was just thinking about the pain. I'd thought about suicide in the past, but never in a way where I'd have done it quickly. I've always thought about ways that would have meant I'd suffer pain. But at that point, the car off the edge of the cliff was the only thing I could think of that would be a painless way of going. The only solution I had to stop the pain I was feeling was to die.

My daughter was around ten at this time, so she'd seen my anger before. This time she'd seen me screaming and shouting and storming off out of the house, and I think that scared her, and then whatever conversation she'd had with my wife made her call me.

Being diagnosed with Crohn's disease also gave me the courage to tell my daughter what she'd stopped me from doing with her phone call that night, which made her think twice about harming herself again. She's probably going to be someone that will struggle with some stuff, and I'll need to help her with it in the future.

When I think about what has happened to me, all that trauma that I needed to unpack, I realise all I've ever done is blame myself for all of it, even though I know deep down, rationally, it's not my fault. This is where the violent outbursts would start – losing my temper, I'd see a wall and I'd walk past it and grind my knuckles against it to take the skin off to see the blood. It was like a way to release my anger, but only hurting myself. I never put two and two together and realised it was self-harm.

I still have the outbursts, but because I've so little energy, I might start screaming and shouting but then I end up just wanting to fall asleep on the sofa, because I'm so exhausted from it.

I'm struggling more now than I was back then because I've realised it all now. The Crohn's disease has put everything into perspective, but all at once, all in one go. When I talk about it, I'm mentally and emotionally all over the place, because something jumps into my brain and I've got to say it so I don't forget about it, and then I've got to go back to where I was. That's pretty much how I am all the time – so when I speak to counsellors or the doctor and they ask what I want help with, I tell them I want help with everything, but I need guidance to figure out where to start.

I think I'm more emotional than I am angry now, just trying to understand why all of that happened to me. I can't imagine putting a child of mine through any of that. It makes me question what type of person I must've been, or am, for so many people – family, people I thought were my friends who bullied me because of people I was related to – to treat me like that.

That's where the self-hatred has come from: constantly looking at people and thinking, 'What are they seeing? How are they portraying me compared to my way of portraying myself?' I really struggle to feel good about myself. I'm not sure I'll ever think I'm a good man. I've tried loads of different things – I even tried setting myself a challenge of doing something good, something to help someone, every day, such as open the door or carrying bags for someone, letting somebody out at a road junction, stuff like that, and even then, I never feel good about myself. I don't know how.

If somebody comes to me and they're struggling, I can talk to them, I can help them, but I can't help myself. I brush my own problems under the carpet by doing something else. How am I supposed to deal with it? I feel like I've got ten, maybe fifteen years before I even get close to figuring this out.

But then I ask myself whether I've even got that long, with having Crohn's disease, so I find myself rushing into things now because I don't know how long I've got left to be able to do things.

I don't know if the Crohn's is going to kick up a gear and be really severe in a year or two, so I'm constantly saying yes to things, because if I don't do it now, I don't know when I might be able to.

My wife relies on me a lot for mental stability, as well as physical help, and when I look at what she's been through compared to me, she's had it so much worse. So I brush my stuff under the carpet, because it's more important to help others than to help myself.

I do want to be able to accept that the anger problems I have now are a result of something that happened to me in the past and make the physical and mental connection. Attempting to get some counselling is challenging because there are so many different organisations out there who can help, but you get lost in the system. It's difficult. I did have a great counsellor through an organisation called Breathe in Cardiff, so I reached out to her again recently, but there's a three–four month waiting list. It's a big challenge to cover that period of time before I, or anyone else, can get help when we don't have any friends to turn to, because we never let people see that side of us, not unless they're really close to us, like my wife. I don't want people to look at me and think I'm weak.

Seeing the opportunity for the Three Peaks Challenge with the Tough to Talk charity, there was no way I was going to miss it. I gave myself the challenge that if I complete it, help the charity, and help myself, I'm going to look at doing something like a sponsored skydive for Crohn's and Colitis UK. That charity has inspired me.

I've lost track of accomplishment; I don't know what it feels like anymore. I'm always looking for it by helping other people out, but by doing all of this stuff, I'm never really dealing with the stuff that's made me the way I am today.

There are times I find myself questioning everything I do, to the point that I actually wrote a poem about it, called "Arguing With Myself". It talks about how I'll wake up in the morning, and in the shower I'll be questioning and imagining what's going to happen during my day.

I'm thinking about scenarios that may happen in an hour, two hours, three hours, because I have to know, to plan, how I'm going to react to situations, especially if someone might be physically confrontational with me. I've got to have some sort of inkling of how I'm going to react.

When I die, I want people to be able to come upon a situation in their life and think, 'Carl once mentioned something about that.' I want to have a long-lasting effect on people, so they never have to feel the way I felt. I can't fix everybody, but I want to be able to talk to people who are struggling and dig down into my pit of knowledge and wisdom and be able to say, "I've been in this situation, and this is how I dealt with it; maybe that could be a path for you."

REFLECTIONS

REFLECTIONS

FOUR

FATHERHOOD: DAN

I'm founder and owner of a small business that specialises in video production. I'm a dad, husband, and an enthusiastic bike rider who rides for the views and cake rather than the speed and the trophy. I love going out and being in nature and open spaces to look at life from different perspectives.

I've always been a passionate small business owner, someone who's very keen on connecting and helping people by using video. Another important aspect about me is that I am a proud dyslexic. In my eyes now this is a superpower, alongside a level of insatiable curiosity and optimism. I used to hide it, as I'd find it hard to disclose my dyslexia and the sort of issues I had, because my school years were between the 1980s and 1990s. Identifying dyslexia wasn't a big thing back then, nor was it supported by society as it is now. Being a proud dyslexic lateral thinker is a gift and I believe is the reason that I'm a particularly good visual artist and storyteller.

I've always been an anxious person, while being optimistic, which I think is a trait of many business owners. I think about things always working out well, but I can also have a tendency to overthink them. I sometimes worry and second-guess things, which can result in going over fifty alternatives of the same sentence in my head. I tracked this back to when we were doing our celebration event at A-Levels; I was about seventeen and the school were giving out funny novelty awards. One of the prizes was "the person with the most PMT,[1]" and I was chatting to my mates and heard the prize giver say my name.

This feels like the starting point for me, when I had enough self-reflection to see that others noticed I had mood swings, triggered by my neurodiversity. I'm an emotionally driven person, whose passion can be fiery, but I'm also very lovely, supportive, and caring at the same time. These emotions and conflicts happening in my head were all fine and manageable, and I was comfortable in my own skin.

In my thirties, I was growing another business, which was a media design agency where I was collaborating with another director that I met at university. I ended up leaving that business because we both looked at life in a unique way and I was keen to pursue work around e-learning and creating learning video content. The other director was a graphic designer by trade and was keen on brand design, so we agreed to go our separate ways.

The separation ended up being a twelve-month cycle of passively aggressively not wanting to be there, which then ended up getting a bit more intense, where we continued to agree to disagree, which was very unproductive. He ended up buying me out of the business, and it was the best thing ever for both of us because we matured and left our university student lives behind us.

Within a matter of a couple years, we had both settled down in relationships and become dads. When we worked together, we were still partying like we were twenty, but it was time to grow up, as we were in our early thirties and embracing adult responsibilities.

I set up my current company and it was a big transition. Selling my share in the previous business was like letting go of my firstborn child, because I'd put my heart and soul into growing it. I love the fact that it's still growing in the right direction, and that I and my previous business partner had made the right decision to go our separate ways.

We left amicably and we've maintained a friendship. I could handle that kind of anxiety because it was healthy anxiety.

When my wife and I conceived our second child, my business had been growing over the years, and we had our beautiful daughter, our firstborn, who was there when my wife and I got married in our mid-thirties.

Approaching our forties, we were on a fast track of building our family; everything was all sunshine, beautiful and romantic, everything worked and was moving in the right direction. Then we went for our twenty-week scan and found out our son was diagnosed with a heart condition. This is when my world went dark, really. I remember it vividly. Being with a consultant and hearing them explain how this is a rare heart condition. We were completely confused, because we'd thought it was our exciting twenty-week scan to find out what sex the child was going to be and all those types of things, and instead we found out this devastating news. That translated over to the next week and the doctors saying, "You need to abort because we don't think the baby is in a position to survive."

At this time my business was doing well, and we'd booked a nice all-inclusive fancy holiday before my wife knew that she was pregnant. With this news, we still went on holiday, which my wife and I couldn't really enjoy, but I was able to drink, and I drank an awful lot. It felt like the only way to suppress all these anxious feelings rising within me.

We used the holiday to think about what our decision was going to be. We went back and forth, and we came back with the decision, which my wife really pushed for, that we needed to get a second opinion, as their prediction might not be true. How did we know what they were saying was true, as he was so small during that period in the pregnancy? We went back and spoke to a different consultant, told him the situation, and he said, "Look, there's a chance of what we're diagnosing, but we don't know. The heart is smaller than a grain of sand, so how can we be sure?"

My wife and I then optimistically said, "Let's go with the odds that it's not," and decided against the abortion, continuing with the pregnancy.

There was also an intervention where my wife had a CT scan so they could look to try and find out more about the relationship between Josh's brain and his heart. Risk was always there, and the risks ranged from abortion to learning difficulties. All these various positions were not the things that we wanted and certainly not what we went into our twenty-week scan thinking about.

The darkness had set in at the first consultancy due to the acknowledgement of what it was, and after that it was hard to believe fully that things were going to be OK. There were various breaks in the clouds and rays of sunshine, and my wife and I worked together to stay optimistic and positive.

Fast-forward to Josh's birth, which was traumatic, as there were issues that resulted in my wife needing to have an emergency C-section and all the stuff that surrounds that. Josh was moved into intensive care, which was our very first experience of it all.

I was trying to deal with everything by myself, as my wife was getting over her operation. Once she had recovered she was on a ward, but Josh was still in emergency care.

I was between the two, and then finally Josh then got out of the emergency care and was taken to another ward for children with cardiac problems, which meant he could be monitored. I remember one instant we were waiting for the consultants to come round to give an update, and you could see them at other people's beds and "Oh, they're coming to us next," but they wouldn't, they'd go somewhere else and then somewhere else. This frustrated me; we had to wait for over seven hours for the update. As I'm somewhat of a fast thinker – others would say impatient – those seven hours felt like seven days.

After about a week, things changed. Josh's condition got better, and we knew that he was on the right track and he was getting stronger.

I remember the moment when the clouds really did split and the darkness came off us initially. It was when the doctors said, "Actually, he's OK and he can go home." I wanted to do a dance, but I knew all the other parents in the ward were feeling the same as I'd felt a day before, so you have to hold back that joy. This news was only a moment of release though, because after that they said, "Look, this is the situation, you know Josh will always have to have cardiology support. It'll always be part of his life." We then got into different pieces of information, went into more detail, and the consultant had lots of meetings with us and some highly intelligent people – doctors, nurses, surgeons. There were massive amounts of information which we were trying to decipher and understand.

We needed time to process everything; we needed time and then we got back to the hospital team. We'd had this ray of hope and sunshine, and left the hospital thinking, 'How are we going to do this? How are we going to tackle this?" We had our daughter who was healthy and happy, but she needed our support as well. She didn't understand it all. I went into solution mode, which is what my strengths are; it's who I am, how I work and why I like to work for myself. I tried to support, understand and learn what all these medical professionals were telling us, which made my anxiety so much heavier. Deciphering this information to relay to our family and being translator was very tough. I wanted to learn but didn't want to learn. I was torn with consuming all this complicated information and a desire to help my family.

We finally met Tommy, who's Josh's ongoing consultant, and he is an amazing guy – really kind, down-to-earth and can put things into plain language we can understand. He'll just say, "It's OK. We need to do this," rather than using Latin medical language which left my wife and I asking, "What are you talking about?" and "Is that good or bad?" – which, admittedly, was often my question. I feel like I'm in a position now where I could write a *For Dummies* guide to cardiology.

The kind of condition Josh has is one where he had two holes in his heart and a common valve, which meant that there was leaking within the heart that needed surgery. He'd been evaluated by the surgical team, and they suggested that the surgery would be performed when Josh was around age four or five. We thought, 'We're OK for now, so let's park it.' And that relieved an element of pressure and anxiety. This was in February 2020, before we heard the news about the pandemic.

I'd just got back to focusing on my business and nurturing my other "child" that I'd created. I look at businesses as children because you do need to love and nurture them as much as possible, so they grow and flourish.

When COVID hit, this forced another layer of pressure and anxiety. The next couple of months things got quite dark, and alcohol really took over to the point where I was thinking I needed support. Luckily, I reached out and got support through the NHS, although the support didn't feel right. I was drinking obsessively, like many people were in lockdown. There was this culture in lockdown where it'd be 11:00 am on a Tuesday and people were on furlough and you could phone someone up and say, "Oh, yeah, I'm sitting in my hot tub having a cocktail," and it was acceptable. That didn't help, as I had this dark cloud hovering over me with my son's heart condition. It was tough, and I tried to fill other parts of my life with DIY projects. I built a garden wall that, unfortunately, collapsed, which was a real shame as I thought it was going to work and give me something to focus on. This was a good lesson learned: focus on what you're good at. I'm good at making videos, and bringing in builders who are good at building walls is far more productive than thinking that I've now got newfound skills because I've watched a YouTube video.

I was drinking during the day, and I knew that it had gotten bad when I started hiding my drinking. I'd drink in the garage. I'd sometimes go to the studio to get work done, stopping off on the way to buy a few beers, then go and drink them, pretending that I was working when I wasn't, as there wasn't any work to be getting on with. I'd send a couple of emails trying to keep the business going. Luckily, we had existing client work, so the business wasn't folding. I was in a position where I could keep it going, but because we didn't have the volume that warranted me working to the level I was *saying* I was, I was using this as a way to hide my alcoholism and the real pain of anxiety.

I wanted to hide it from my wife and the kids, although at the same time I was thinking, "I need to do something about this." Some friends were starting to see what was going on, but they didn't see me all the time because we were in lockdown. Eventually, I'd become somewhat of a manic depressive, where the alcoholism and the anxiety took things to that next level.

I'd spoken to the NHS in the past about my mental health and had tried antidepressants years ago. They hadn't really worked out, and I realised medication wasn't the right answer for me. Exercise was. However, getting out on my bike, I'd ride, then I'd then go and drink, because I could justify it since I'd just done a sixty-mile bike ride. I'd tell myself, "I can now drink whatever I want." All these justifications were to give myself permission to drink every day.

I got to the point where I didn't want to become an alcoholic. I was telling myself, "This isn't right. I've got a family that I need to look after and protect." It was negatively affecting my life, but it was hard to face due to the simple fact that I felt happy when I drank. It felt like it brought some fun and happiness to my life, like when I'd read the kids stories and make very funny voices when I was drunk. I wasn't paralytic, but I certainly wasn't really thinking about my actions. My children didn't know anything about what was going on because they were too young to understand the difference between funny dad, silly dad, drunk dad, and grumpy dad. I was just Dad. My wife could see certain aspects of my behaviour, and we'd talk about it. She was also in a dark place, so she wouldn't obsess about it, and she'd sometimes drink with me. She's not a massive drinker. She went really inside herself at this period. We're opposites; I'm fight, she's flight, but she went into freeze mode, and I went into alcohol, which went beyond positive opposite attraction. It went to a negative space where we couldn't find common ground and would argue.

We started to think about divorce, and this brought up childhood trauma of my parents getting divorced, things to do with my dyslexia, self-doubt, paranoia, self-sabotage, just an overwhelming number of negative things going on in my head. The only way that I could deal with it was to ride my bike, eat cake, and then go and drink a couple of pints, which appeared socially acceptable, then get drunk when I got home.

The real turning point was when I went from beer to spirits and I realised, "I don't like who I am. I don't know what I'm doing." I was forgetting who I was and what I was doing. I got to that point quite quickly and said, "No, I have to do something about this now!"

I reached out to the 111 doctors advisory service, telling them, "I'm in a dark place. I need support. I'm starting to have suicidal thoughts." I hadn't taken any action, but the anxiety was getting to the point where I was having physical panic attacks that really hurt. I've never felt pain like it from a psychological and physical perspective.

The doctor prescribed me a mild dose of antidepressants after I was referred to a GP, but as we were still in lockdown, I had to speak with the doctor over the phone. My dosage increased as my panic attacks increased. The antidepressants did work to suppress a part of the pain and mental illness I was feeling.

They also helped to reduce the amount of alcohol I was drinking but didn't stop me altogether. My kind of alcohol culture was one of a social nature, but I was certainly drinking to forget rather than drinking to celebrate. Alcohol ended up becoming a horrible friend that I couldn't get away from. It was this relationship that I couldn't hide, and so I reached out to Turning Point, which is a local Leicestershire charity for drug and alcohol rehabilitation.

I enrolled in one of their programmes, which were good. Between my first dose of antidepressants and my support worker, things started getting better. It didn't take away the doubt, the dark cloud and the uncertainty of the diagnosis from Josh's twenty-week scan, which was the root of my suffering from anxiety and stress.

We were still spending a lot of time at the hospital and had some challenging conversations with Josh's surgeon. At the time, unfortunately, they were trying to clear their patient list before moving the children's cardiology unit to a different hospital. Culturally, from an organisation perspective, I could see massive issues in front of us, because the Glenfield children's cardiology department was amazing and nationally renowned, and it was moving. The staff were all in an uproar, protesting and saying, "We don't want to do this, we don't want to move," and we were told children's cardiology were moving to the Leicestershire Royal Infirmary.

We initially thought that Josh's heart operation was going to happen at Glenfield, until it was cancelled due a chronic chest infection – fortunately, not due to COVID. With all the different elements that were going on, and still being on antidepressants as well as trying to manage my alcoholism, I was so relieved I was finally getting some good support through the counselling at Turning Point.

I heard from a nurse that the hospital needed to increase statistics because they were low on heart operations, so they were trying to fast-track my son. We went in for what we thought was an initial consultation to start rescheduling his operation, and the surgeon told us, "Oh, you're booked in for next Tuesday."

Suddenly the world went black again. I got angry with the surgeon and the NHS in general. Their lack of compassion and empathy for my family's well-being was becoming very frustrating. All I wanted was to protect my family and keep my business going through the hardship of the pandemic and all these other challenges that were going on around us, which created more stress because we felt that we were fighting a system that I didn't want to fight.

My anxiety put me into fight mode, and I ended up trying to fight the people who were trying to help us – which just didn't help. Once I delved deeper, I found out that I was in the right about my concerns; not that there's a right or wrong, but they had their targets to meet.

Luckily, the operation was postponed again due to my son's ongoing chest infection, which was the best thing and the worst thing at the same time, as we were back in waiting mode. I literally felt like I was back in the waiting room from the twenty-week scan where the darkness started, and it was kicking in again.

My alcohol levels increased again, and I started smoking marijuana to try and suppress all the darkness whilst managing all these different moving parts. Fortunately, we were getting back on track work-wise, winning new business. I was wearing a mask, going around pretending to be this happy, positive person in front of clients. Putting on a front, then going home and hitting the bottle to deal with the fact that I'd worn this facade. I didn't want to be there, even though I was enjoying the work. I didn't want to do it because I just wanted to support and defend my family, and be there as the father figure for my son, which I didn't believe I could really do, as I felt so much fear.

Finally the cardiology team moved to the Royal Infirmary, and we were one of the first families to go there. We had ended up with three cancelled operations before the surgery happened, and although things were getting tough, I was building resilience, learning from all of the challenges, and understanding how to tackle it in the right way and not fight.

The cancellations were due to Josh's health, but one time surgery got cancelled an hour before it was due to start. My wife and I had our war paint on; we felt like we were in the trenches, and we were ready to go, to face the storm. So then to be told about the cancellation, we were back to ground zero. It felt like a kind of *Groundhog Day*.

Eventually Josh had his operation, and it was tough, one of the hardest days of my life, especially towards the end of waiting over four hours of surgery, which felt more like forty years. I remember trying to be positive, playing the joker, trying to support my wife. We went for a walk around Leicester, trying to look in shops and just in a daze as we walked over eighteen thousand footsteps. Then we started to panic that they hadn't phoned us as planned. We arrived back at the hospital wanting to find out what was going on and ended up sitting in this waiting room with other parents, watching the mixed emotions of joy and despair. It was surreal, seeing all the other parents, their sad eyes and body language, and just the overwhelming feeling with no one being able to give us an answer for why things were delayed.

Due to the cancellations, I'd managed to rebuild a positive relationship with the surgeon, and by then I was somewhat glad and understanding that he lacked empathy. At the end of the day, he's a surgeon and he just needed to do his job, which he does very well. He's an amazing heart surgeon. I wouldn't give him a medal for offering emotional support, and I certainly wouldn't open up to him, because he wouldn't know how to deal with it, and that's not his job. Unfortunately, mainly due to COVID, there weren't any nurse liaisons to help us, so the experience certainly didn't feel supportive and caring.

When we spoke to the surgeon, he started with his Latin lesson in heart surgery, to the point where I saw this passion and excitement in his eyes, but I didn't really know what he was saying due to sleep deprivation and stress, so I interrupted to ask, "What's going on?" He said, "Oh, we've had to do things differently, which I've never really experienced, and with this being a rare case and …" I had to interrupt again: "Just stop! Is he OK?"

He then replied, "Yes, he's OK." And I responded with, "Well, that's fine, because everything you're saying is just going over my head, and now we can start to relax. Now I can go and sleep. Can you tell us what you just told us again once we've both slept and maybe draw us a diagram?"

Then a sense of relief started kicking in. We knew that Josh was OK, although he still had to have five or so days in intensive care. This was traumatic because we knew he was getting better, but it was still hit-and-miss, as he'd had major heart surgery. There were times when other kids didn't survive, and seeing that was dark. I wanted to try and help the parents, but you can't help because you're focused on your child. It felt like I was standing in a queue behind them, thinking to myself, "Am I going to be served that same lunch?"

A couple of dads and I ended up having conversations, breaking down the process and the information, sharing the emotions we were going through, and I really wish, with hindsight, that I'd had more of those types of conversations. That's why I want to share this now. Talking therapy is so important. Sharing what you are going through may be traumatic and emotional, but it's another positive step towards building mental strength and well-being.

Thankfully, we were told the intensive care wires could be taken out, and that was one of the most positive wins in my life. Within an hour our son started getting colour in his face again. Then he started eating some beans on toast, which sounds so trivial now, but it was such a relief.

The bright lights finally started coming through the dark clouds that I'd carried for over three years since the twenty-week scan. My optimism and the real Dan were finally coming back, and it wasn't that I had to pretend that things were going to be OK; this was based on genuine evidence now.

I'm generally quite pragmatic and evidence based, although if someone that I trust says things are going to be OK, I trust them and then I'll go with it. That was all the evidence I needed. From that point on in his recovery, it was like looking at how a runner bean grows so fast, where you can practically see the plant growing. We'd been told that he would need to stay in hospital for about seven days after intensive care, and yet within two days he was jumping around and thinking he was Spiderman again.

Unfortunately, we had to tell him he couldn't be Spiderman because he had to stay on the ground for about two months. Due to all the cancellations delaying surgery, we were now in a position where our son could talk and walk, so looking back I'm so glad they all happened, because he was just a baby when we first went into Glenfield. He now had an element of independence, which was so positive because he could tell us when he was hurting or happy. When he was discharged, it was amazing, and we went home, finally feeling supported with a real sense of resilience and gratitude.

With all the uncertainty I carried, the counselling that I'd had along the way was incredibly positive and the lifeline I needed. I've continued to get private counselling, which has been a great investment; talking therapy really helped me get my life back on track.

I was finally in a position to go for a bike ride because I wanted to go for a bike ride, not because I could go to a pub at the end of it. Finally, my psychology was changing for the better. If I did want to go to the pub, it would be to relax and enjoy life, not to hide and suppress any negative feelings.

When Josh was in recovery, I suddenly realised that all the risk-aversion consultation that we had received was typical of the NHS. This made the experience far worse than it should've been. Yes, they have to be cautious, but the lack of empathy and compassion was very hard to stomach.

Depression is an easy diagnosis for the NHS to give, along with a quick serving of medication, which in my case I don't feel is a bad thing. My wife was also diagnosed with depression and prescribed the same medication when she *wasn't* depressed and had very different mental illness symptoms. That's not to say the NHS medication and counselling doesn't work sometimes; it did support and reduce my symptoms. It wasn't the best solution for me long term. Talking therapy helped me to build my own resilience, positively reflecting on the learning I'd gained from all those hard knocks. It was the main thing that got me out of my long-term anxiety.

I still have a manageable level of anxiety, but I'm no longer suffering from panic attacks. I wouldn't recommend it, but I self-medicated myself off the antidepressants. The NHS didn't reach out to offer me any support to come off them, I just gently reduced the dosage. The antidepressants didn't work for me as a long-term solution, but they helped me along my journey, and they're a lifeline for some people. I'd recommend them if you need release – and don't fear them. I was hesitant, as they felt taboo, making me feel like a failure. When I got the right dosage, they worked, and I was able to see through the darkness ... but the things that really worked for me long term to tackle my anxiety was to talk about my feelings and to do physical activity. The talking therapy helped me so much that now my best mates and I talk about mental health openly. We talk about when we're feeling depressed or anxious and all of that stuff I wouldn't have done before. When we go through these chapters in our life, we come out the other side feeling stronger.

At times, the suicidal thoughts I had throughout this journey presented themselves as a feeling of complete worthlessness, where whatever I did wasn't right. I was so paranoid, feeling like my marriage wasn't working and I was an irresponsible dad by drinking too much. Everything that I was doing was wrong. I was in such a vulnerable position; I couldn't really see a way out. My panic attacks started to get so bad I wanted to rip my skin off, and in those moments of complete illogical nonsense, suicide seemed like a possible answer.

My wife was amazing and was, fortunately, there to support and help me through those dark times, and when I came out on the other side of the panic attacks, my rational brain came back into play and said, "NO! Those aren't the right kind of emotions. Those aren't the right actions. This isn't the solution, there is a better way." I told myself to go for a walk or go for a bike ride because it was the best way, and sometimes I used alcohol, which would suppress the anxiety.

If you're feeling like this, I'd suggest reaching out and talking to people who aren't your friends or family. Don't rely on your friends and family to have the answers. Reach out to the NHS; despite their problems, it is a caring system, and we have this amazing public health service to help us. Especially if you're at that rock-bottom position, they will give you help if you need it.

If you can afford to pay, I'd recommend getting private therapy, because you can get the help far quicker, and you can get that release that is far better than any form of drug or alcohol to relieve these mental pains. My wife and I also had marriage counselling and we're now back on track, rebuilding our relationship. I feel married again now.

When you feel the pain coming in, don't be scared to acknowledge it, and act before you get to the point of mental breakdown or burnout. It's so easily done. As a man, one of the hardest parts was that I felt I needed to be the hunter-gatherer of our family. I wanted to be the protector. I wanted to be the father figure that found, deciphered and translated all this information. If I'd reached out for support in the initial stages when I was pretending to be strong and wearing a mask, it would've helped me so much, and I probably wouldn't have gotten to the dark points that I did. I feel strong now, confident that I can talk about my problems. It's not a taboo subject anymore because I've learned about my mental health and being open to being emotional.

I've learned that's it's OK to cry if needed.

And most importantly, it's OK to be happy.

---

1. PMT – Pre-menstrual tension. (This was a popular gag used at that time to poke fun at people who got angry quickly and without perceived reason.)

REFLECTIONS

REFLECTIONS

REFLECTIONS

FIVE

NARCISSISM: BEN

I'm forty years old, a self-employed management consultant, and I've lived at home with my mum since the beginning of 2019. I became homeless after splitting up with my fiancé and I converted a cabin in the corner of the garden into my workspace, creating my pit of iniquity and a home for myself.

By 2013 I'd been through a really tough time. Relationships had left me in a vulnerable place with pretty low self-esteem. Work was tough and I'd do anything for everybody and have nothing left for me.

I got angry a lot, drank more than I should, but wasn't an alcoholic.

I'd grown incredibly lonely; my dad was getting ill, and my brother had moved on with his life. My career was all right, I made decent money, was saving for a house; it wasn't a bad life. I just kept meeting people who'd use me, belittle me, and just generally take me to pieces.

Whilst on a dating site I matched with someone who had a profile image of a glass of wine the same size as her head. I chose to crack the joke "you're absolutely my sort of person if you can drink that amount of wine in one sitting, well done!" With hindsight, I realise that was a terrible mistake.

Becca and I clicked immediately, met up within twenty-four hours, and had a fun time. Things happened rapidly, and looking back, there were an unbelievable number of red flags.

I introduced her to my housemates, and she criticised the state of our home. My friends were not impressed, and I made excuses for her prickliness and over time all was well.

She'd recently split up with her fiancé as he didn't want kids and she did. I wanted kids so we both wanted the same thing. After three months she asked me to move in, even though he was still living there. I thought it was a bit strange, but I just went with it, moving in a week after he moved out.

We argued constantly during the first month, then I met her best friend, Veronica. Shortly after meeting Veronica, Becca dumped me and said, "You're not my type, I don't want to see you anymore." I was in shock and found myself inexplicably on the phone to Veronica attempting to justify my behaviour, "I don't get what I've done or why she's being like this. And I don't get why I'm on the phone to you!"

I messaged Becca to try and gain understanding. Eventually she replied, "I'm sorry, I just wasn't feeling it." After three weeks of no contact, she got back in touch, saying she'd changed her mind and wanted to give it another go. I agreed and moved back in.

With hindsight I see the mistakes I made. I've gone over these stories so many times to try and make sense of things. They've become so familiar. I feel them rather than remember them.

My overwhelming feeling from the beginning of the relationship is abject chaos, a constant push-pull of being good enough and not good enough. Speak with my friends, then don't.

She had a stressful job which meant late nights working, a job that took up a lot of her time. Although she made decent money, it got in the way of us spending time together. Sometimes we'd fight because we'd arrange to spend time together, then she'd get a call and have to deal with it. I understood her career was important, but so were we.

Sometimes I felt I was in a position of "The ex is gone; you'll slot in nicely. No change needed." I remember feeling there was no room for me, and I'd ask myself "What's wrong with me? I'm a decent bloke. I try and do right by you and be what I'm supposed to be" but I felt like a lodger. She tried to kick me out, and I'd ask, "Why? Let's communicate, Let's *actually talk* about these issues instead of just having blazing rows." Each time she'd shut down, turn, and walk away. I know now that is withholding, but back then I didn't know what it was.

As blokes, we get frustrated and angry, and at the time I didn't know where to put this anger, which made me angrier. And this really annoys me about how both men and women both misunderstand men. We have testosterone running around our veins which is worse than crack cocaine, and if you put a man in a situation where he's under pressure for long enough, he's going to go pop. Testosterone causes us to lash out and be angrier than we intend to be. For years, I'd been getting worse in terms of my anger, how I responded and dealt with it, and it came from this place of frustration.

I didn't know who I was, why I felt the way I did, or how to cope with all the things I was experiencing. I didn't even know *what* I was experiencing, so with all this confusion I'd get angry, hit floors and walls to the point where I'm now missing a knuckle on my left hand.

I did everything to hurt myself because I felt better when I was hurting. I'd get this great endorphin rush and when I headbutted walls, doors, or anything I'd get the feeling of, "oh yeah, that's better". It would snap me out of the funk, changing how I felt. It would interrupt the cycle of anger that was building up.

Now I understand this was self-harm, but back then, I thought I was just being angry and lashing out. I didn't want to be angry or feeling mad at people, didn't like being upset or feeling that rage. I think many men feel the same way. They don't know where to put that anger once it starts building up, and when you've got somebody constantly jabbing at you, it's not easy to deal with.

When I was angry, Becca would tell me "You're getting angry. I can't talk to you when you're angry," which would only make me angrier. I just wanted to communicate but I couldn't, so I'd walk outside and release the rage because I didn't want to be angry around her, or anyone. I wanted to calm down and not present this image of "You're one of those angry blokes." I didn't want to be that. That wasn't who I was.

Thoughts that I was a terrible and evil human being deepened my sense of shame about how I was handling what was a very tough situation. My self-talk was horrendous; I absolutely hated myself. If I were saying all this to another man, I'd expect him to punch me. I destroyed myself with what I was saying.

Becca and I reached a plateau of how things were going to be. She'd go out and see friends, which I'd encourage, as I was happy she had friends to socialise with. She'd go on work do's, attend meetings at all hours, telling me it was needed for work. I'd been cheated on before and started smelling a rat thinking she might not be where she said she was. The screen on her phone got smashed and I offered to get it repaired. I sat on the stairs at home with the repaired phone in my hand with thoughts of "I don't have the right to look." I knew it was wrong, but I had a look and found evidence she'd been cheating on her ex for years and had been cheating since we'd been together. One message really cut me to pieces because she referred to the 'leg jerk', aka orgasm, all the time. I fell apart as I'd been cheated on more than anyone else I knew. It's one of the reasons my self-esteem was in the toilet.

I remember sitting there crying with the phone in my hand thinking, "It's happening again,", "Why am I doing this? Why am I putting myself through this? Why is it always me?" I didn't realise at this point I'd been targeted.

Becca came home and found me in a state and it's one of the few times where I saw genuine concern from her. I came clean and said, "I looked through your phone and found messages I wasn't expecting, but sadly was. You cheated on your ex and now me."

She seemed terrified I was going to leave her, that she wouldn't be able to have kids and or present this image of being a successful woman holding down a happy relationship. Back then, I thought it was genuine upset and terror that she'd hurt me, that she felt bad for what she'd done. She talked me into staying, even though I'd proven to her I was untrustworthy after that point. I'd done the unthinkable and that day that the relationship broke beyond repair.

The levels of toxicity increased, and the double life that she'd been used to became impossible. Something also broke in me that day as I lost respect for myself because I stayed. I could've moved out; things could've been different. I could've lived a happy life and gone in a different direction. But I didn't. I stayed. She told me these other guys were out of her life. Sadly, I believed her because I genuinely saw her as my last chance. I thought that nobody else would want me because there was something wrong with me.

A few months later, she told me she was moving to Derbyshire to renovate and live in her grandfather's house. No warning, no nothing. I had two choices: go with her, or rent our current home off her.

In a state of shock, and my self-esteem so far in the toilet, I decided to go with her, telling myself that it'll be fine. I'm a capable guy, I'll find a new job but whilst negotiating with my employers to hire me long distance they said no. It screwed me, but we made plans and moved up to Derbyshire.

My parents would be thirty minutes away instead of two hours, so I supported my mum who was struggling with dad's dementia. We moved to into two flats which hadn't been touched in thirty years. Living in the upstairs flat, we sorted out the downstairs, then switched. I invested tens of thousands of pounds in terms of materials and manual work, and enjoyed knocking through walls, clearing the site, and smashing up cast iron bathtubs with sledgehammers, as well as the decorating. The problem was the place belonged to her and her brother, so I had no say in anything, even though she'd tell me it was my home, and I did have a say. I suggested turning the two flats into a family home as we we're going to raise a family there, which backfired whenever there was an argument.

With her friend, adopted sister, and ex-lover, Veronica lurking in the background, constantly sniping at me about my politics, work, my presentation, anything you can think of, there was this constant refrain of Becca and her friends being the most important thing, with me coming second to all of them, especially Veronica.

I knew my place, accepted it, because Becca had had some tough times. She would regularly make it known my family and I were not welcome. If my mum and dad, even my brother, were around, there was always a face like a smacked arse, and especially if Veronica was there. It was horrible, and we all felt unwelcome in what was supposed to be my home. I was still feeling like a lodger.

Becca would bitch about her friends, and then be nice as pie to their faces. She'd be assassinating their character, and although I had criticisms of some of them, I didn't agree these insults were warranted. I didn't understand why she did this, but now I see that creating unequal or misrepresented views of people gave her control over how everyone interacted around her. It gave her a position of power, which she craved. She wanted to control my perception of her friends and prevent me getting close to them. She would tell me what she wanted me to about them, rather than have me find out for myself. The fact that I knew so much eventually became a problem for her.

After Becca and Veronica stopped speaking for nine months, Becca and I became close. We had a real relationship, went on holiday, and had a lovely time. We still had problems, but for the most part we had fun. It was my birthday gift to Becca, but all the way through the holiday she was on her phone. Checking her phone again, I discovered she was messaging another bloke, whilst we're on holiday! I thought we were getting closer, and yet there's another man on the scene. I never challenged her on it, she never told me, I just accepted "this is my life, this is what I'm worth."

After our holiday she told me, "I really want kids." I've always wanted to be a dad; my dad's amazing, so I loved this idea. She struggled to conceive, so we did some research and found one of the biggest causes is stress. Her job was kicking her arse, she was constantly complaining about it, so I suggested she take a short career break.

She quit her job making sure I never forgot I suggested it, and two weeks later she's pregnant. We're both over the moon, ecstatic, feeling amazing and meanwhile, Becca's aunt had been secretly communicating with me from America asking if Becca and I were going to get married. Becca is the first woman I'd ever met that I wanted to spend the rest of my life with, so, her aunt and I cooked up this plan for me to propose using a ring that belonged to her mum, which her aunt had. Her aunt sent me the ring and I created this night out with all our friends. Sadly none of her friends turned up, so me and my friends went out and I proposed in a restaurant in front of everyone. Becca was suffering with morning sickness, so wasn't feeling her best, and when I proposed, she was mortified. I could see by the look on her face, but she said "Oh, go on then." Everyone thought she was being funny and ironic, but I knew it was a case of "If I have to." She was cringing, she didn't like being the centre of attention anyway, but at the same time she was mortified that I'd asked her to marry me. I gave her the ring which barely fit due to her hands being swollen with pregnancy. We never discussed marriage or the wedding. She was my fiancé, and I felt it was a case of "I've done it to make you happy."

Shortly afterwards, my dad was taken into a care home as his Alzheimer's and dementia worsened. It took him seven years to die and that absolutely kicked the crap out of all of us, especially my mum, who nearly kills herself dealing with it. My brother did what he could, but he lives far away. I was closer, so I supported Mum through it all. We'd struggled to get Dad into the care home, until I told the community nurse and social worker that, "If you don't do something to help my mum, she's going to kill herself. And I'll probably do myself in because I'd have lost both parents. Do not kill my family." I then burst into tears and that's when they realised they'd miscalculated the seriousness of the situation and agreed to take some pressure off us all. It was easier, but not easy, as we watched my dad slowly disappear and die. It was horrible.

Gavin, my first son was born in April 2017, just before dad died. It was a traumatic birth as he got stuck around the perineum and came out all blue and floppy I don't think there is anything that traumatises me more. He gets injected with Vitamin K, wakes up with a good scream and I almost collapsed with relief. Becca's in the tub, worn out, bless her having given birth to a nine-pound baby boy. The midwife passed him to me first and said, "Here's your son" and it was nothing but pure love. It was amazing. To meet my little boy under those circumstances, to know that here's a little dude that I can support, nourish, and cherish, be there for him like my dad was for me, to be that hero, I thought, this is it, yeah, this is life. All this we've been through; things are going to get better. You get to be a dad. That's cool. My dad wasn't perfect, but he was my hero.

Gavin was in hospital for about a week in the special care baby unit because he got an infection inside the womb on the way out, hence why things were so tough. Becca stayed with him, and I was shuttling between the hospital, home and work trying to sort everything out. My mum was an absolute star helping us out as much as she could around Dad, as did my brother. We get home and that's it: I'm a dad. She's a mum. We're learning about bathing, nappies, screaming in the middle of the night. We learn about breastfeeding, sore backsides, no sleep, baby food, no time for yourself, and we learn about no time as a couple. And then on top of it all, I learn about how pretty much everything is my fault. Again, the messaging that I'm just not good enough.

It didn't take long after her pregnancy for Becca to start feeling like her life was over. She couldn't pursue a career or drive her two-seater sports car anymore. She couldn't go drinking with her friends, go out partying or just disappear off to places and do things. She couldn't be the person she was, and the most convenient person to blame was me. Things got even worse when we argued, and I started retreating. Gavin kept us together, and he was about two or three months old when I felt like we we're done. I refused to admit it to myself, but I started dreaming of what life would be like without her.

At five months old, we introduced Gavin to my dad and the look of joy and love on Dad's face was priceless. Dad was getting worse and couldn't remember who people were, He'd have angry moments, and was difficult to be around. The hardest part being around somebody with dementia is when you leave, they ask why you're leaving, they want to know where you're going.

In September 2017, dad died in the home, and none of us were there. I still don't know how I feel about him dying without us being there. When it came to Dad's funeral, I attempted a speech as I've always been a speaker, a showman, Mr. Jazz Hands. I stood at the front, said my piece, and dissolved into a crying wreck. Becca's mum died when she was eighteen due to brain cancer and rampant alcoholism, so she understood losing a parent. She was there, and I could see she felt genuine emotion and compassion for me. After losing my dad, I stopped caring. I was there for Gavin as best I could be, but I just felt like he wasn't my boy, due to all Becca's cheating and because a previous girlfriend had cheated on me and gotten pregnant by another man. I started switching off, packed all the sadness and grief away, telling myself "This is your life now, mate, deal with it."

As time went by, I got angrier. My friends and their other halves had become friends with Becca. 'The WAGs'[1] were having kids at the same time and bonding. Becca was bad mouthing me to family and friends, and yes, there was a lot of valid criticisms of my behaviour back then, and I was my biggest critic. Switching off the numbness got harder, and six months after we had Gavin, Becca says, "I want another kid." My reaction was "Have whatever you want. I don't care." She was happy, so the next, and last time, we had sex, she gets pregnant.

Around that time, Veronica's fella Paul, who was ridiculously close to Becca, starts having trouble with Veronica; she kicks him out and he comes to stay with us. Becca fell pregnant with Robert around this time, and I got it into my head that they'd cheated, and Robert was his. Thoughts of "He's got to be my kid. We had sex. Deal with it, Ben, you know he's yours." Being in a very dark place, I started forgetting I had a son.

Work wise, I was involved in politics which was absolute hell. I went through several jobs because I was so stressed, and eventually stopped caring about work. I was doing alright, and it was work that kept me going, helped me to find some self-belief; then I lost my job.

I started freelancing to try and get some money coming in but a side effect of constantly being undermined, belittled, and torn apart is you can't concentrate or deliver. Society says, *"As a man, you must go out, be the hunter, the gatherer, bring in the money, be the rock, the steady influence, the sure person." I couldn't do that. I was ruined.*

In late 2018, I started work as a 'high falutin' Marketing Director, Mr Intelligent, making all the high-powered decisions, but I'd be sat in my office crying with no idea why. I thought "I've had a hard day, let's have a cry" and that it was healthy to cry. To a point, it was. I didn't understand why I was so upset or what was wrong with me. Why did I feel so numb? Why was I drinking more than I should? Why was I getting angry around my friends? Playing computer games with me was hell because I'd throw my controller across the room or smash stuff, all with a little one running about doing his thing, *That's the worst I'll ever feel, scaring my kids because I'm angry. Beats everything I've ever done.*

Becca didn't have much free time, but what she did have she spent on her phone gaming and avoiding me. And to be fair, I was the same because I didn't want to be around her. I resented her and didn't like who she'd become, how she made me feel about myself.

Our second son Robert arrives in August 2018 weighing 10lb, even bigger than Gavin. He also got stuck with his shoulder in breach. Becca had to get out of the birthing pool and started walking across the room with Robert's little face poking out of her nether regions as she gets over onto the bed. There are some things you can't unsee. Then a specialist comes in, snaps Robert's collarbone, twists him around, and he's out. Job done. He's born with a broken collarbone. Both my kids came into the world in trouble. And scared.

Robert looked a lot more like me, so I knew he was mine, and I just loved him so much.

Late 2018, I had completed three months of therapy which I'd been referred to by my doctor. Becca and I started to talk again, and it felt like we were heading in the right direction. After my birthday in December, I get the urge to look through her phone again and found more evidence of cheating. I felt despair, anger, and just thought "Fuck this! Fuck me! Fuck life! Fuck it all!"

With two kids Becca expressed feeling like she had to take care of them alone. But I'm there. Everybody thinks having one kid is hard, and they think that until they've had two kids, especially when they're pretty close together, and still in nappies. With money worries on top of everything else, things started spiralling out of control.

I didn't understand what pregnancy does to a woman in terms of body image, self-image, confidence, or lack of. The total destruction of the person they used to be because their body has completely changed. Some desires have changed, others haven't, and I didn't recognise that, like most blokes don't. Nobody sits there and takes you through this stuff. Looking back now, I can see that Becca was desperately unhappy with who she'd become. Being isolated and cut off from people; she was struggling with life as a new mum. She had to make it work and did the best she could to cope, as well as coping with me and my issues.

Being a new dad, I didn't know what that really meant. I'd also just lost my dad, and work was getting beyond the pale.[2] As a couple no constructive conversations were happening, no understanding about where we were, what we were doing, and other people, including Veronica, her family, and friends started interfering.

I put my hands up, I was obsessed with work because the thought of being a new father scared the crap out of me. I'd finally realised it's real, it's happened. I'm a father to these two small humans. I'm supposed to care and do all this stuff, but I didn't know how to be a dad. For Becca that wasn't enough. She wanted me to do more, be more, be healthier, stronger, and I couldn't be the person she wanted me to be. The difficulty I had in coping with that, was it wasn't just my actions or failures that she was commenting on, it was me. She came to the conclusion that as a father, I was a failure. She separated my role as a father from my role as a person, which I later found out was an actual psychological thing. As a fella, she had already decided I was lacking in many ways. She found me weak, feckless, and couldn't tolerate me. She wanted to train me up to be better man, a better father, and as a fella, that's pretty tough to cope with, especially as a father, who had the disgust and the disdain from her friends.

I'd derive my self-worth from work. The person I was at work was bullish, confident, a go getter. At home I was whipped, and soon my work life met my home life. I hated myself and thought I was a failure as a father, so why bother? I've got a family, a house, a flash car, all the things, and I just accepted it.

Much later I started reading prolifically about men's abuse and how men's persona works in 2023. I consume social media content like crazy. One of the things I saw was that men are told to accept what they get: Just put up with it, that's the best you can get. You're not worth anymore. Don't get above your station. Don't think you're anything better. You're just like every other bloke out there. Put up with what life deals you, otherwise you're a whingy little bitch. It's that sort of toxic masculinity idea that creeps in and that's the view I had of myself.

If I could go back and have a word myself, I'd say, "Right, you and me, we're going out for a beer, have a chat and you're going to come out of this a different bloke because you are worth it. You've got so much to give. Your boys want more from you." I could be a better man for Becca now than I was back then, because I've had a chance to heal. I've had a chance to look at myself in a different way. Whereas back then I just couldn't do that.

Becca got back on the alcohol quickly and I'd find empty wine bottles around the house. I'd drink with her occasionally and she'd tell me I wasn't interested in the boys, her, or our family. In my heart and in my head, I was screaming "God, I'm so interested in this family, in this house, in you. But you don't want that. So, why am I going to sit here forcing something on you that you don't want?"

She constantly wanted, and got attention from other men, and if I tried to give it to her, it wasn't enough. She wouldn't accept compliments from me, nor my attentions physically or emotionally, so I switched off.

Shortly after Robert was born, I became unemployed for a couple of months. We worried about money. We've got two toddlers in a house that's halfway through a refurbishment and we've run out of money to carry on. It was a tough. I found another job, but I was getting into debt. My savings and nest egg I'd been putting aside disappeared because I was giving her money each month. I didn't know where it was going. I didn't ask. I didn't want to know. I just wanted her to leave me alone, because anything she said to me was shaming and demoralising. She told me it was Post Natal Depression. I believe some elements of it were, but it was a heightened version of what she'd been doing all along.

Things got was worse with Veronica around due to their codependent relationship. Looking back, I think "How did I ever feel that was acceptable?". It's difficult to speak about it in meaningful, rational way because I'm so far removed from the person I was back then.

Having two kids, watching her decline and struggle with being a mum and taking on the lion's share of parenting, which was obvious she didn't want, was tough. She wanted to get back to work as soon as possible because she wanted the life she had before we met. She resented me being the father of her kids, for putting her in a situation where she was now poor.

My new job as Marketing Director started out interesting but soon became an absolute mess. I blurred the lines, played politics, did all sorts of things that I shouldn't have done. Looking back now I think, "Ben, you idiot, why are you doing these things? Why did you take those steps?" I'd be one of the first to arrive and leave because I didn't want to be at home.

I'd arrive home and sit in the car trying to rustle up the courage to go in. One night after I'd been sitting outside, I went in, and Mum was there. With my cheery face on, I said "Mum. Great to see you. Are you alright?" We had a cuddle, and I turned to Becca and said, "I've got a bit of work to do, so I'm going into my office." All I needed was thirty minutes to decompress so I could step up and do what was needed. But I wasn't allowed that time. Becca was so frantic because she'd been with the boys all day. She lashed out at me, "You come in from work and the first thing you do is go and hide rather than say hello to the kids."

One night, Mum said, "Ben, I can't do this anymore. I'm having panic attacks coming to your house and leaving." That broke my heart. Seeing the look of my mum's face when she told me, "You're going to hurt yourself, if you don't deal with this" I didn't register how bad it was. Mum was the only person who witnessed and experienced Becca's abuse; and was the first person to tell me, "You need to think carefully about your future here."

Mum loved being grandma and wanted to be friends with Becca, to support her. Becca claimed my mum as her own so mum would stop by regularly to help with whatever she could. Becca's family life wasn't great in many ways and she didn't get the help and support she needed from various agencies.

Not long after Robert arrived I started having suicidal thoughts realising "I've made a massive mistake. I'm with a woman who doesn't love me. She loves the idea of me but not the reality." I'd cringe making love and being intimate with her because I felt I was being used. I'd been used as a reliable 'piece of ass' before, both mutually welcomed and unwelcomed, but in this situation I wanted to spend the rest of my life Becca, even though she's telling me, "There's something wrong with you. You're mentally ill, you've got real problems. Either you sort out your mental health or we're done." And again, I agreed with her because I'm the one with the anger issues scaring the kids. It was horrible.

After Robert's birth in August 2018, Becca was playing more

games on her phone, drinking more, and taking more money off me every month. I didn't know she was on a gaming app, spending hundreds of pounds, whilst chatting to other men. Her first night out with her new friend Katie, I told her to have a wonderful night and waited up. She stumbled in drunk at 5am looking as if she's had her kit off. She vomited on the stairs, and I cleaned her up and put her in bed. I looked at her phone and saw a message from a bloke called Dave "Thanks for an amazing night, Hope to see you again soon." I couldn't believe it. On her first night out and she's already playing away.

I continued with my delusion, gaslighting myself, and I didn't even know it. I became more suicidal, with paranoia, self-harm, and drinking the norm. We were two separate people living in the same house; and I still felt like a lodger.

In August 2019, I found a therapist and told Becca I needed some time. She responded, "In that case, you need to move out, go through the counselling, and do what you need to do." I agreed until my mum made the comment, "Might not be you, sunshine. There's stuff going on that you need to think about carefully." Becca had poisoned my relationship with my mum by that point, so I was questioning my mum, and my brother.

Packing up all of my things reality hits like a hammer. I cried like I've never cried before, and the kids come up to me. Robert asks, "Daddy, are you alright?" I collapse on the floor and tell him "Please go downstairs and be with your mum." He runs off crying and that's one of the hardest memories I've got because his daddy was in pain and he was confused; only to have me tell him to "Go away, kiddo. I love you. But you can't see this. I don't want you to see this."

Downstairs the boys stood either side of Becca. They looked scared, confused, and didn't know where to put themselves. She looked at me and asks, "Have you got everything?" I replied, "Becca, I don't want to leave you, or lose my boys and my home. I want to be with you." She dismissed me and I left. That was one of the hardest moments in all of this, the realisation that it's done. I'd been fearing and worrying about this moment for years. I knew it was coming, could see it getting closer.

After being in therapy, I invited Becca to resolve our issues together. She resisted, then agreed. Within ten minutes of our first session, I was bawling my eyes out, "I'll do anything. Just make it stop, I can't cope with it anymore. I just want us to work. Please, I'm begging you."

The therapist saw the contempt and the dynamic, stating, "Couples therapy is not right for you." I continued my sessions with him and was happy and curious. I enjoyed the process of figuring out what was going on within me and learning about psychology. For the first time I considered I might be able to feel free of the way I felt.

Living with Mum, with time to myself, free of being abused every day, something started changing and I started having this back and forth with myself, "What about me?", "What about you? You don't know what you want? What do you expect? Oh. Yeah, but…. What about me?" The voice was there consistently.

In the beginning of 2019, I decided to confront Becca about Dave. She denied it and said "If you're accusing me of cheating Ben, you need to ask yourself when I have the time to go cheating! Get Real!" Totally gaslighting me, and three months later, I was in a full-blown nervous breakdown, but continued working on commercial contracts for business.

In May 2019, a colleague started showing an interest, and I found myself reciprocating. We started having an affair, but I didn't know she was under 24/7 surveillance by her ex-husband. I had feelings of guilt, but at the same time excitement because somebody's *actually* interested in me. Sharing our mutual situations, I felt a connection and didn't feel alone. I had a space to go, and it was therapy as much as it was sex. She would listen, ask questions, and wanted to talk to me. It was amazing and I loved this feeling. It was tempered by the idea I was watching a slow-motion explosion of everything I wanted and cared about, but Becca didn't want me and enjoyed watching me slowly burn in front of her. My anger started ramping up.

In August 2019, the ex-husband of my mistress broke into her home whilst I was there. He stole my wallet from downstairs, marched upstairs and started attacking me, whilst I'm starkers.[3] She's screaming, I'm defending myself without violence. I told them to sort themselves out and he kicks me down the stairs. I grabbed my stuff and left. I knew I could've killed the guy if I'd lost it, and I wouldn't have stopped. I didn't want my kids to have that man as their father, so I kept that part of me locked away.

As a kid my temper would come out to play regularly. It caused me problems and I'd hurt people, so I swore I'd never be that as an adult.

The husband shows Becca the footage and she calls me and shouts "You cheating bastard! I know exactly what you've been doing. I've seen the messages, the footage!" I didn't know what to say other than "Yeah, I've been cheating. I'm sorry." It was the strangest thing. I thought I'd strongly deny it or get angry. I didn't hide the affair. I wasn't deleting messages. I'd leave work to see her and stayed late, so I clearly wanted to be caught. What was left of my stuff Becca dumped at Mum's, and said, "I never thought *you'd* cheat."

Being around my mum made me feel worthy as a man, and I started to see what she saw. Becca had torn me apart, programmed me to be her slave and whatever she wanted me to be, so she could discard me when *she* chose to.

Becca spent two years making sure everyone knew about my affair, trying to drive a wedge between me and everyone I knew. A lot of the people I thought were my best friends, my social support network, just abandoned me. Four weeks after everything came out I attended my best friend's wedding. I didn't want to go, but my friend and his partner told me I absolutely had to go; I was part of their family. I turned up, crept in, and sat behind my other best mate, Gary at the back. I tapped him on the shoulder and said, "Alright mate!" and he looked at me disgustedly and said, "I'm not judging mate, I'm just disappointed." This triggered my stress levels so badly I couldn't speak.

I'd worked on how to handle these triggers and so handed him my phone, with a page on the Mankind Charity website which described how to tell others you're being abused. It listed all my behaviours others had witnessed: the anger, frustration, the social distancing, problems at work, the inability to look after myself, and the falling apart. He looked at me disinterested, dismissive and gave me my phone back. It was clear that he and many others didn't want anything to do with me, except, one friend, Matthew who tried to talk to me throughout the day.

I wanted to tell people what had happened, but this was not the time nor the place. This burning desire to talk meant I had to find time to myself, to calm down. Being surrounded by couples and families with their kids, was torture. I should've politely declined, but I was in denial. With moments of being the guy that can take anything, soldier boy, as I call myself, I kept telling myself "I'll cope, I'll be fine.' And I wasn't fine. I began to shake with the stress of it, got funny looks from others, so after the reception I gave the bride and groom my apologies, told them I was leaving. They thanked me for going. Friends I'd grown up with, one's I'd been through thick and thin with, dismissed me. To have them all publicly shame and humiliate me in front of those I loved and cared about was incredibly painful. I got in the car and started crying, and it wasn't long before I was thinking of how to kill myself. I'd had enough.

Just before the wedding, after the affair had come out, my brother and his daughter were visiting mum. I was in such a state, I told my brother, "I've done something terrible; I've had an affair. I've ruined my life." My brother replied, "Oh, when you said you've done something terrible, I thought you'd killed somebody." I responded, "I feel like I have." He told me we'd talk later. I laid on the floor for four hours and couldn't get up. I just lay there looking at the ceiling, telling mum, "I want to die. I've had enough. I can't be here anymore living like this. I can't feel this anymore." Things no parent should ever hear.

My mum sat with me holding my hand, talking to me. She was incredibly brave. In therapy I'd learnt a few tools out how to manage and cope with what I was feeling. They kicked in, everything disappeared, and I asked myself, "What have I got to live for?.." Looking at the ceiling I reeled off this list: doughnuts, beer, attractive women, fast cars, then computer games, my kids, my family, friends. Bear in mind, this was before the wedding, and I had my friends. There was travelling the world, seeing unusual things, wondering if aliens exist. Volcanoes were on the list because I love volcanoes. I reeled off things I had to live for, and I came to the logical conclusion I there was no point in killing myself. A big part of it was my friends who I thought would be with me through thick and thin. They'd proven that before. I called my therapist, and I said, "This has happened. I'm in a really bad way what do I do?"

He replied, "Well done."

That totally threw me. "What do you mean?" I asked.

And he replied, "You called me. That's the healthiest thing you could've done. Well done."

After the call, I could tell myself, "I can do this!" because at the very least I've got my friends. Finding out at that wedding that I'd based my strength on my friends killed me inside. It really hurt, so that's why on the way home from the wedding I wanted to kill myself. I scared myself and pulled over into a layby and cried. I put on some music, shut my eyes, and fell asleep. I'd stress myself out so much I passed out. When I got home, I told mum what had happened, she could see why, so I spoke to my therapist again.

Becca continued to gaslight me with requests of sleeping together, anger and niceties. I wanted to see the kids as often as I could, and it was a weird limbo state. Everybody was in a bad way. My message never changed: I wanted her and my family back. I wanted to go home, make up for what I'd done, move forward because I was *still* in denial.

Negotiating the terms of our relationship I moved back in to see if we could fix things. We stayed in separate bedrooms. I'd set up a business alongside my political activities, providing a campaigning platform for people. Becca hated my involvement in politics, because she wouldn't tolerate failure. She'd tell me I was wasting my time, should be working, making money for us. "You're putting us at risk because of your pet projects." She was right, my business didn't last long because I was too traumatised.

2020 arrived along with the pandemic. Work was horrendous. I was blamed for the dismissal of a sex pest, and a new guy was hired to get rid of me. On top of everything at home, my boss was making my life hell. I was made redundant before furlough kicked in, so I was jobless again.

For three months I was back in the family home, Becca tried to be considerate, and avoided being completely self-centred. There was visible effort being put in, she was seeing things from multiple viewpoints and considered I have my own goals, life, and directions. She admitted in messages and e-mails that she'd abused me; then she gave up.

Things became toxic again. She'd tell me, "I'm amazed you're still doing that business. All the others failed." Everything went completely wrong; I packed up my gear in front of the kids and left.

For six months after leaving, I saw the boys once every six weeks and Becca didn't make it easy. Mum and I would go over and help as much as we could. I'd do maintenance on the house, building trampolines for the kids, whatever I could be dad and a good co parent. I'd do my best but most of the time I was disallowed, disavowed, and generally just treated like crap.

I realised I was being edged out and she'd made it clear the kids were hers, yes I was the dad, but she made all the decisions. Things became even worse if that was possible. Her resentment of my business working infuriated her as I wasn't taking orders from her or anyone else. She had this attitude of "Who do you think you are?," something she had been projecting onto me for months.

The kids had nowhere to sleep at Mums, and I didn't have any money yet to be able to do my part in terms of being a co-parent. I'd left that relationship with £1500 and two broken cars. I was rebuilding from scratch. She constantly asked for money, and her relationships were causing me problems, namely with Veronica. I knew I didn't want to have Veronica around my kids and Becca started to threaten me with non-molestation orders.

I received letters from her solicitors ordering me to, "stop contacting our client."

I asked, "How the hell am I going to see my kids? I want to see my kids. I want to be their dad. How am I going to do that?"

They replied, "Get representation."

They knew I couldn't afford representation, so I had to figure out how to get access to my boys. I didn't know who to speak to, there was no cooperation, until she suggested mediation.

I was dead against it because I believe Becca is a narcissist, and from the research I'd done, narcissism and mediation is a very risky manoeuvre, often re-traumatising the victim. I caved because I wanted to see my boys. We had our orientation calls, which resulted in me exploding into tears, confirming to the mediator this wasn't a clever idea. If you want to go to court, you need a piece of paper that says that you tried mediation within a given amount of time beforehand. I was told I'd receive a piece of paper stating mediation wasn't right, or safe, for me. I was relieved because I knew it wasn't.

When the letter arrived, Becca demanded to know "How have you got that? What have you said? What have you done?"

I told her, "Becca, I'm not safe around you. You're my abuser."

When she heard that, she reacted as if I'd slapped her. She couldn't accept the truth of the situation, so she resorted to threatening me with the police and solicitor's letters again.

Finding a settlement in court would require between £15,000 and £25,000 pounds. My therapist told me the waiting list is a minimum of eighteen months just to get a first appearance in court, so either I got my application in and wait or try and compromise. He was pushing for the latter.

I wanted to see my kids at weekends, but Becca wouldn't allow me in the house or co-operate with travel, so the boys and I spent the day together at play centres, everything always on her terms.

Through therapy, my recovery, and the research I was doing about abuse, how co-parenting works, and the law, I was becoming aware of what was and wasn't possible, as well as the good and not so good ideas. I realised Becca was trying to control me again. I told her, "I'm not going to be under your control again. I'm not going to put myself in a position where you dictate to me how I live my life and raise our kids. That was happening in our relationship. You were overruling, undermining and gaslighting me, trying to ruin me. So, I'm not going to do it."

She agreed to me seeing the boys. We needed a compromise, so she asked me, "What do you recommend?" I'd downloaded some co- parenting guides, adapted those, and gave her a detailed proposal, informing her it was up for negotiation. Her response was a hard, flat out "No" to it all. Throughout she never told me what she wanted, only what wasn't allowed, which is pretty much everything.

Without my therapist, I wouldn't be here. I would've killed myself. He helped deprogram me with psychodynamic therapy, allowing me to ask myself, "What are my boundaries?" Being able to push back in a constructive way was evidence that I now had boundaries, something Becca hated. With the combination of therapy and Krav Magar, a form of Martial Arts developed for the Israeli Defence Forces, I had the perfect combination. I was able to put my rage somewhere; and this is the most brutal martial art there is, and I absolutely smashed it. Talking with people who would sit down and just shut their beak and listen also really helped me. I still had some of my old friends who stuck by me and listened. They'd tell me to visit for the weekend, I'd tell them what happened, we'd make food, go for walks, and I'll always be thankful. I could never explain what it meant to me to have their support.

Having people who are able to listen is priceless, because most people aren't equipped and don't have the emotional strength to be able to cope with it. They feel like they should say something when in fact they shouldn't. Listening is all we need most of the time. Most people really find this stuff really triggering, difficult to deal with, so I can understand why they don't want to listen.

I had the trifecta: I had therapy, physical exercise and self-belief kicking in, with people who can listen. Running my own business also gave me something to focus on. It gave me purpose because I could no longer be dad. I became a businessman and my identity shifted giving me somewhere to put my energy. Many guys who go through what I went through, have nowhere to put their energy, so they turn it inwards through drink, drugs, violence, sex addictions, gambling etc. They find some way to destroy themselves by turning that energy inwards. And we can't, we've got to put it outside of ourselves. We've got to bring it out and shape the world in a positive way. A toxic environment turns a person toxic. My situation proved that. I wasn't in a good way and being in a toxic environment just made it a million times worse.

My biggest concerns were making sure I had input on decisions about how the kids are schooled, healthcare decisions and how they're brought up.

I just needed some safeguards, some boundaries so that I could be sure that I wasn't going to get abused again.

This was the major mindset change. When you're in a situation like this with kids, most people put their kids first. They think that's the right thing to do. And it isn't. Learning this was one of the things that saved my life. Yes, kids are important, but we are the most important person in our own life. We must put ourselves first. Our ability to be here, show up, be healthy, to have a life to function, and to be a parent, we need to be alive and capable of it first before we can be there for our kids.

Many people judged me negatively, and I had to get used to it. They'd tell me, "I'd do anything for my kids."

My response is, "Really? You would run yourself into the ground and end up dead, would you? Well, that's a great thing to do for your kids, isn't it? Put yourself in the ground so that you're not there for them."

And they never have an answer, because they haven't lived it, they can't comment from a space of knowing.

It got to the point of no contact, other than me checking on the boys and trying to get access to them. I received an e-mail stating my messages to Becca are harassment and abuse, and if I didn't cease contacting her, she'd call the police. The only way I can speak with her is through a lawyer. I don't have the money to afford a lawyer, or the mental health to go through the fight again. I've set myself a goal of having enough money in the bank to buy a home for me and the boys, and once I've got that in place, I'll put aside a legal fund and fight to get my kids back so that they can come and live with me 50/50 when the time arises.

There's no point in speaking to the police because I'm a man. I can't sit there and say, "Look at the bruises, look at the scars, look at the damage that's been caused me" as I didn't know I was being abused, and wasn't recording evidence. There's no case to stand on in terms of fighting for a domestic abuse situation which means social services won't get involved and nobody else will give me any support.

There are no charities that can do anything. I'm completely on my own with no support. All I can do is talk about what I've been through and help people understand that when men are in a situation like mine, 50% of them commit suicide. They can't cope with the parental alienation, with losing their kids, watching their abuser get away with murder and have everybody believe the abuser is the victim. Men like me can't work, they drink and do drugs. We get violent, and we get angry due to testosterone raging through us. Men who've been traumatised are stigmatised because of that trauma, because of the way we react to it. At no point will I ever sit there and minimise what women go through. Not in the slightest. Women have had hell because there are so many traumatised men out there.

And when we stop traumatising men, we stop traumatising women. It's that simple.

My therapist said I'm a textbook case of how to handle it. In terms of coming out, positively fighting, putting myself first, being positive, and practising radical acceptance about a situation that is horrendous and living with it. I haven't seen my boys in over three years and have lost the most valuable years of their childhood. I think about them every day, and the grief I feel is hell. I wake up each day feeling like a 10-tonne gorilla is sat on my chest.

My mission is to be the best person I can be, to do myself the most justice, to deliver myself the most respect, and in doing so, be the father my kids can be proud of. So that day I get to be their dad again, I'm not who they've been led to believe I am, and I can say to myself, "Yeah, I'd like you as a dad. You're a pretty good choice," then I can find solace.

I've learned to find a space where I can acknowledge, "it's all right. I can live with this." The only person who can fix this situation is me, and I'm really lucky because I'm a smart guy, I'm healthy, I've got a family that loves me, friends that care and I can now get things done. I reach for the stars and the moon, and I'm one of the few people in this situation who actually stands a chance of grabbing the moon and saying, "Right I'm going to have you!" Me and the moon are getting my kids back, because I know if I work hard enough for long enough, and I kick enough arse I can do it. I believe it. And that belief, that hope, is what keeps me going.

I'm sharing my experiences because I want to see men stand a chance of being who and what they can be, so the rest of the world can benefit from half of its population, rather than being treated like disposable consumable cannon fodder, which is how we're treated.

The law, and the societal situation needs to change. The trauma informed movement for me is a massive thing. It's important and needs to happen. But what I'm seeing is a whole lot of anti-male propaganda coming through which I don't agree with. I'm far from a Men's Rights activist, but what I don't believe in is demonising men further because the problem isn't men, the problem is the life men live and most of the time, that life is traumatic. It's hard, uncaring, unfeeling and it hurts them and when they're hurt, they're going to hurt other people, unless they can go through the healing journey.

Telling my story in a coherent way means pain is no longer relevant to who I am. I've put it down and moved on with my life, becoming the person I want to be. I'm tired of being hurt, of other people hurting. I'm tired of negativity, and I want to make it better. I'm a fixer, that's what I do. I call myself the business fixer. I've turned how I feel into a business. I used to be a people pleaser, a people fixer and wanted to go around and fix everybody around me because I couldn't face fixing myself. Now I know how it affects me, because I've had the education, and I've given myself time to heal.

I'll continue doing my part in fixing things until the world is a better place, because it cannot carry on as it is. I hope, and fear, my kids somehow learn this. They're two little boys growing up in a world that doesn't treat men very nicely, and I'm not there to guide or educate them; and I desperately want to be. They're surrounded by people who I believe are seriously problematic, and I know at some point I'm going to have to try and unpick the damage that's done to them in terms of how they're brought up and their value system.

And I'm going to have to live with not being there.

I wake up and I go, "There's damage there, there are problems there." Stuff that's my fault, that's to do with me. Stuff that's not my fault, but it doesn't matter. I've got work to do and I've got every day for the rest of my life to do that work, and I'm bloody well going do it.

---

1. WAGs = Wives and girlfriends
2. Going beyond what's acceptable. Outside the limits of acceptable behaviours or judgements.
3. Totally naked

REFLECTIONS

REFLECTIONS

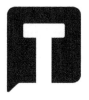

SIX

ANXIETY: JOEL

I'm the lead singer of an up-and-coming band, and I'm surrounded by a loving family and good friends. I'm in good health, and I've suffered from health anxiety since I was twelve years old.

I was raised by two loving parents in a small northern town and had a fantastic older sister. We were, and remain, a close, tight-knit family, and I cruised through early life. I was very outgoing and healthy, played a lot of football, loved going out, meeting people, and being with my friends. I could be a little reserved when meeting new people, but it didn't take long for me to shake that once I got to know them. My childhood was great. While I was happy in general, I started to suffer from what I now know as anxiety; back then, it was referred to as "being nervous". I became anxious about doing what seemed to be little things to everyone else, but they were big in my world.

The big turning point was when I was ten years old. My mum and dad split up. Though young, I remember it very clearly. It was quite an abrupt split, and it threw me and my sister in at the deep end. It was the kind of thing I thought only happened in films; you never think it's going to happen to you. Looking back, I now know it happens to a lot of families, but when you're ten, your whole world collapses. Everything from then on was split: family, activities, family events and Christmas.

In secondary school, when I was twelve or thirteen years old, I started to get anxious about my health. It took over my life for a good three years or so. I was convincing myself something was up with me. It got to a point where I'd tell my mum I wanted to go to the doctor and have a full check of everything to see if there was anything wrong with me. My mum took me to the doctors, but when we got there, she told them about my anxiety. The doctors arranged for me to have some CBT[1] sessions, and although I didn't quite realise how it was helping me, it was good to have someone to talk to.

After I finished school, I went to college and started getting into music. I started playing the guitar properly, playing the gig circuit and writing songs. I'd play all day, every day, and since then, I've found a love and passion for music.

Growing up in a small town, there wasn't a huge amount of opportunity for a young, aspiring musician, but I knew I'd found something I was good at. My sister started posting videos of me on Facebook playing acoustic songs, and the positive reaction gave me the confidence I needed.

This led me to go to Manchester to study music at university. I was keen to start a band, and this was a good starting point. When I moved over there, I was pretty nervous, like most first-year students, and I wanted to meet some like-minded people and experience university life. It worked out pretty well, as the band members I spend most of my life with now are the band members I met in university halls. We were placed in the same dorm by chance – fate.

From the time I left school until my second year of uni, I felt like I had my anxiety under control. I'd been so busy with life, excited by music and new hobbies, that I guess my mind couldn't really think about my health. That was until my second year. I'd moved into a shared house with a lot of people. We were doing pretty standard student stuff – going out, drinking, partying a lot, being around new people, having bad sleeping patterns ... the list goes on. But the switch in lifestyle ended up being a turning point for me. My anxiety peaked and I was at my lowest ever.

The anxiety consumed me again. These thoughts about my health consumed my mind every day. It was physically and mentally exhausting and interrupted the quality of my life. I was so scared of dying; I'd find any reason to convince myself it was happening. I eventually told my family, and they assured me everything would be okay, but it got to a point where I realised I needed to talk to someone about why this was happening to me and try to understand why I was having these thoughts.

I needed more than reassurance and more than someone telling me to speak my thoughts out loud to try to justify them. I was internally shouting out for help, and people close to me were just trying to give me the answers they thought I was looking for. The doctors suggested medication, but I turned it down.

I ended up booking private CBT sessions with David Knight in Manchester. It was one of the best decisions I made. Speaking to a professional you don't know personally is a lot easier than talking to someone you know and love. He didn't tell me the things I wanted to hear either. I completely broke down in my first session. I brought up a lot of difficulties, and David helped me speak through them, something I'd never done before. The deeper issues were the reasons I was experiencing these anxieties, and once I understood the root of it all and my triggers, I viewed my anxieties differently.

With the transition to university life in a big city, and having come from a close-knit community, I believe there needs to be more awareness of mental health in young people, especially when a lot is going on and it's all a bit crazy. The stuff I learned in those CBT sessions gave me a different way of thinking about things and helped me learn how to tackle the thoughts that came into my head and how to deal with them.

The sessions gave me so much clarity and a different viewpoint. I started going to the gym, got a job and was creating music. Eventually, the lads and I moved out of the shared house, so it was just me and the band living together, focusing on our music, and that's when things started to take off a bit. I then moved out to live with my partner, which was great. Life was good. As a band, we took the lockdown during COVID in our stride. We did some live-streaming sessions to keep our fans going and wrote a lot of music, and it worked well.

Fast-forward a few years: we were on tour performing to crowds as big as 2,500 people. Life was fast-paced, and, while my anxiety always lingered, I was able to control it. The morning after our last show, I had a phone call that a close family member was diagnosed with stage four cancer and had three months left to live. Those three months were the toughest three months of our lives. No words to explain it.

A year passed, and my health anxiety started to kick back in. My family encouraged me to book a few CBT sessions with David again. Rather than allowing my anxiety to spiral, I needed to nip these new feelings and thoughts in the bud, understand them, control them and deal with them. David, again, put my anxiety in perspective.

The start of the year 2023 was tough, and I'm taking things as they come, which is what works best for me. I know how to tackle it and how to deal with it now, which is important – if I'd been where I am now a couple of years ago, I wouldn't have been able to separate the anxiety from normal life. It's still difficult – the mind is strong and strange, and if you let it, it'll take over your life.

I'm focusing on my music, enjoying my life as much as I can and surrounding myself with the right people. It's been difficult to speak about my family member, but I think it's important that I do. They were a big part of my life, of all our lives. I think we sometimes avoid talking about people who've passed away, so that we and others don't get upset, but we need to speak about them. It's healthy.

I've tended to bottle things up throughout my life, and it's not done me any favours. Talking to someone about my struggles, openly and honestly, and telling even just one person about how I'm feeling has lifted the weight off my chest.

I've learned to prioritise myself and take at least half an hour every day for myself, unplugged from the world, social media and work. My experiences with my mental health have kept me grounded, and I now feel better placed to talk to others about their struggles and be more aware of other people's signs.

I'm twenty-eight now, and the rule is still the same whenever I get anxious thoughts. I'm a better son, brother, partner, friend, colleague and band member because of it. It's also helped me make my songwriting more real – the lyrics speak truth and I just tell it how it is.

My advice to anyone struggling with their mental health would be to just keep going. Speak out, ask for help and believe in yourself. Find the root of why it's happening and when it does, how to handle it. It's doable, trust me. Remember that you're not alone, you're absolutely not the only one going through it. Look after yourself, listen to yourself – your mind and your soul are different, and sometimes your mind can take over your soul. You've just got to listen to yourself and tap into the real you.

Life can continue in a healthy direction. My anxiety is part of who I am and always will be; it'll never disappear, but I know how to work my life around it, rather than the other way round. It will never control me.

---

1. CBT = Cognitive Behavioural Therapy

REFLECTIONS

REFLECTIONS

REFLECTIONS

SEVEN

CUMULATIVE: KRIS

I'm a lecturer at a local college. I've been in the motor trade pretty much all my life and decided to leave the world of spanners and teach. I dabbled for a couple of years in the world of personal training, and that kind of teaching just didn't really pan out for me. I had a passion and a love of sharing knowledge with people, and that's what got me into teaching. I came straight out of industry and went into it.

Things were good when I met my current wife, who had also struggled with mental health issues. The career change was a step in the right direction for me, and I've been where I am now for four years. Things were going in the right direction for both of us personally, and we were both happy.

Everything was looking good; we had a marvellous future ahead of us, great plans, and she decided that she'd come off her medication and see how she was. Unfortunately, she took a little bit of a decline and became depressed. I took that as a personal attack on me, because I kept thinking to myself, 'Well, what am I doing wrong? Am I doing something wrong that's stopping you from being happy?' I couldn't understand, because she had a great career, loved her job, home life was good and we both had great prospects. We'd made plans to get married and had other plans too, so I was left wondering, 'What is it that's stopping her from being happy?' We had a few disagreements, and eventually she decided to go back on her medication, and after a while she started feeling better, and I felt happier because things were looking better.

The point where it really hit home for me, where I was really struggling with my mental health, was, as cliché as it might sound these days, during the first lockdown in COVID. It wasn't anything to do with the fact that we were cooped up indoors or, like a lot of people said, they felt like their freedom was taken away from them. It was more the teaching-from-home element of working, having to learn to teach remotely after only just starting my career in education. The college I was working for put out an email to say there were free distance learning courses that members of staff could take alongside our normal teaching. We weren't face-to-face as much with the students, so we had more time. I thought, OK, it's a free course, and it gets me another qualification, potentially. I investigated which courses there were, and I chose one that was about understanding mental health because of what my wife was going through and her struggle with her own mental health. I thought, 'What a great way to help me understand why she feels the way she feels and why.' I wanted to understand why she was in the position she was in and learn how to support her.

I started doing the studying and learning all about the different aspects of mental health and what types of mental health issues people could face, like stress, anxiety, depression and all the different things associated with mental health. As I was reading through a book, all I kept thinking was, 'This is me'. The picture that was being painted of how people behave or how they can be in terms of their demeanour or their general mood was a perfect picture of me. I thought, 'Oh my God! This is exactly how I am.' Reading about the different kinds of stress and depression, I ended up saying, "This is how I react to certain situations. This is how I put myself forward.

This is the way I am." I then got to thinking, 'But why? I've got all this stuff; I've got a home, I've got a future wife. I've got a great career now, and so why is it like this? How have I got to this? How? What? Why am I now struggling with my mental health?'

As I started reading a bit further into it, I referred myself to the doctors to get some help and advice. I spoke to a therapist, and it turns out that I've been struggling with my own mental health for a lot longer than I thought. We ventured into it, we looked at different areas of my life and what my childhood was like and past events that potentially led to me being the way I am. I'd got to a point in my life where I thought, this is who I am, and I just accepted that this must be normal. Getting stressed easily is normal for some people, and this is how I have been and always will be.

When I look back through my whole life and my history, there are a lot of things that have led to me being the way I am, and I wasn't OK with that anymore and I wanted to do something about it. Going through the journey, I feel like I've started to move towards the end of it. I've got more motivation. We've got a lot of projects on the go at home, a lot of stuff that's keeping me busy but also keeping me active and keeping my mind busy. I've finally started to live out my dream of competing in men's physique, as well as motivating myself to better my career, earn more money and start doing more of the things I enjoy. I've highlighted the fact that I'm not the sort of person that's happy sitting still. I need to be doing stuff, and that's helping me to deal with it as well. When I look back at the things that have happened in my life, it's only now that I really understand why I got to the point where I was.

The thing I want to get across is the fact that some people might be struggling with mental health but not actually know about it. They might be suffering from depression, stress or anxiety or some other form of mental health struggle, and they may be in the position that I was in, thinking, 'Well, this is just me, this is just the way I am.' Unless they talk to someone, they are just not going to know. For me, it took that moment when I was doing that study course and reading that book to suddenly realise that I hadn't noticed it. It was quite bizarre and profound, really, to get to that moment of "hang on a minute, I'm not OK" and have it really hit home that I was struggling with my mental health.

Looking back and understanding my mental health issues, I realise it has affected the people around me. In general, I feel I'm quite a nice bloke, a decent stand-up guy, but there are those moments when something triggers my anger and I react. I'm not overly aggressive, but because I'm six foot three, a fairly big guy with tattoos, a lot of people find me potentially intimidating. So when I react to something in an aggressive manner, a lot of people see it as worse than what I think, and so I've had to train myself to rein that back in a little bit and rather than react to a situation, take a step back and try handle it differently.

I read a book a little while ago called *The Chimp Paradox*, and it explains that we've got two sides to our personality. A chimp, which is the irrational side, the reactive and unreasonable side. Then you've got the human side, which is the rational person, who'll think about a situation before they react to it. That book was quite helpful, and I highly recommend it to others. I started reading it and I said, "Wow, this is clever," and it's a simple concept really.

The professional support I received was when I got referred to counselling by the doctors, and the most important way it helped me was to be able to look back over things in the past and try and highlight the triggers, the things that may have led to me being the way I am and struggling with my mental health. Everybody goes through tough times in their life. Everybody goes through difficult relationship breakups, and there are lots of different things that people go through, and when I looked back at my childhood, I realised it was very, very difficult. But I in no way believe my childhood was worse than other people's.

My mum and dad had no money. My dad was and still is an alcoholic and quite a horrible guy really, who filled our childhoods with broken promises, lack of love and emotion, and genuine fear. As much as he's my dad, and I do love him, I used to dread the time that he came home. My dad used to drink at a pub that was literally right at the end of the road where we lived, and he was so lazy he used to park his van right at the end of the road, go to the pub, and then after a couple of beers he'd get in his van and drive home and park outside the house. When he got home, he would drink even more. I remember there were so many times I used to go to the front bedroom window, look down the road and I'd see his van was there, which meant he was going to be home soon, and I'd start dreading his arrival. I'd go hide in the bedroom and try and keep myself out of the way.

My parents stayed together for a long time, until I was about eighteen years old. When I look back at that relationship, I understand it to be poisonous, and I think mum and dad should've split up long before they did, but they tried to keep it together for the family, which is admirable but at the same time probably did more damage. Growing up, my dad was quite physical with me sometimes, and I remember there was one time I got myself in a little trouble and my dad decided to headbutt me, and there were other situations like that, and that possibly could have triggered my anger outbursts. When I look back at our childhood, my sisters and I were clearly an inconvenience to my dad.

When I was about nineteen, I got involved in an issue with some neighbours about the way my dad was. We got into a fight, and I ended up with quite a big blow to the head after being jumped by another person. Again, you could look back at that and think, 'Well, was there some sort of damage? Is that what caused it?' It was things like that, trying to establish "what triggered it?" and then being able to recognise when I get to the point of feeling like I did back in those days, and then doing my best to try and manage it.

When I look back at my work history, for example, I used to get stressed all the time at work because I was constantly on the go. I was just so busy and I was very career driven, career focused, and I've always worked hard and always will. That's the work ethic I've always had. I'm a grafter, not lazy like my dad. I found myself getting to the point where I was getting stressed at work, and I was coming home with massive headaches and migraines because I was making myself poorly just through trying to better myself. Everyone has got aspirations to some degree, and everybody's got goals. They all want to get somewhere, there is something they want to reach, but sometimes they can be a little bit unrealistic, and sometimes if you're trying so hard to reach that goal, that itself can become stressful.

I went through a messy divorce because I was stupid enough to get married at twenty-one years old. That was a rocky relationship with a very messy breakup. There are lots of different events that I've gone through, that other people go through, and you find yourself isolated. When I look back at these events I always wonder, why was I so alone through those times? I had no one to turn to, I had no one to rely on to help pick me up. When I've gone through breakups or when I've been heartbroken or things have gone wrong, there was no one there. When I lost my garage business, for example, which I had for a few years, it got broken into and a lot of tools were stolen. The building had been smashed up and trashed through the jealousy of other people. I was alone through all of that, and I started heading on the wrong path, drinking lots and just destroying myself.

There are lots of different things that can happen in the past, and being able to highlight all these things is extremely important because in some respects you forget about it because you don't think about it daily, but it'll always be there in the back of your mind. It's very difficult to try and brush it under the carpet and just say, "Oh no, it's fine. That's in the past." But it still affects you; it affects you years down the line and you don't realise it.

That's why it's important to be able to open up and talk about those things, and sometimes it's good to speak to a stranger, to speak to someone you know is not going to be judgmental, someone you've never met before who you know in a professional sense. They're able to help you look at the potential triggers, and they can give you coping strategies and mechanisms to help. Sometimes that's better than talking to people you know because the people that know you might not necessarily tell you the things you need to hear. They might tell you the things you want to hear because they know you as a person. Whereas a professional person will just be upfront, and they will be honest with you because they're not there to judge you; they're neutral.

The coping strategies and mechanisms I use when those past traumas raise their heads is to try and put a positive spin on those events that have taken place. Those negative events in your life have potentially made you a stronger person, and even though you don't feel like you are, you've gone through those things and you've come out the other side and you're still here. You've still got people around you that care; you've still got a life to live whether you've got friends and/or family. Focus on improving how you feel and improving the way you are in terms of being able to cope with certain things; you might find that that will enhance your life, and you'll have people around you and, more important, people that care.

For example, if the wife says something that's annoyed me, rather than standing my ground, getting into a negative conversation, I now walk away for a bit. I calm down, and if I feel like I need to discuss a certain thing, I'll try and have the discussion. Taking a breath and walking away to calm down gives you the opportunity to put perspective on it, and then you get to ask yourself, "Do I really need to talk about this? Probably not, because it's not really a big deal", or "That really did bother me, so I am going to try and discuss this, and I will approach it in a positive way rather than just being angry." It's those different coping strategies that have certainly helped.

I don't believe I've ever experienced any stigma or discrimination because of struggles I've had in the past, because I've been quite open with people at work about the fact that I've struggled with my mental health. I was really shocked at how many people at work do struggle with mental health, and it's a massive thing at the minute, and I do think COVID has influenced it. There is still that stigma attached to mental health, but because I'm quite open about the fact I'm on antidepressants to try and control my emotions whilst I'm still dealing with these things. I hope that eventually I won't have to use them, but I don't feel quite ready because I'm still studying for my teaching degree and I'm still doing a lot of other stuff that would put a lot of pressure on me, which makes me feel like I don't want to come off the medication yet. It is taking the edge off; it's helping me to process a lot of stuff.

Being open about the fact that I'm on medication, I've realised there are still a lot of people that see having medication for your mental health as a negative because you end up not caring about other stuff, which is not true. It's a chemical thing, it's something going on within the brain, and it's an imbalance of hormones, which people don't see or want to see. They don't see antidepressants as a positive or a way of having a safety net to process everything and to get help. They don't see that I'm being positive, proactive, and trying to do something to better my life, his life, their life. Some laugh at you and say, "You're just on your happy pills", and if you find yourself in that situation, you must shrug it off. I've had disagreements with people at work. There's a particular member of staff who does certain things that are very questionable, and sometimes when you question them, you get a little bit heated, and one of the things that's been said to me is, "You need to go and take some more of those happy pills." So there is still stigma around it, but it's not as bad as it used to be.

Mental health has been hard for a lot of people, and it's getting better, particularly through certain avenues within the government that are addressing many of the issues. There's also the fact that I have seen lots of kids struggling with mental health, particularly this year, as there are a lot of kids coming through college now that have got mental health issues, and because I'm in the position I'm in, being on medication, I have more empathy for them. I have a better understanding of people that struggle with mental health, whereas years ago I might've been one of those people who are continuing the stigma. But you can't, because you're not helping people that are struggling with real problems by doing that.

I've been prioritising self-care now for several years by training in the gym. The gym has always been a place of solace for me, but the last couple of years I've taken it a bit more seriously. Last year I entered my first bodybuilding competition, and I placed in two competitions, so I was happy with that. It's also giving me another focus, and even though I'm not competing this year because I want to focus on getting my teaching degree done, my plan is to step back on stage again next year. Blokes need hobbies; guys always need something that's going to keep them busy. I have my motorbikes and the gym, the two things that make me happy aside from my family. They are the two things that help me to deal with certain things. If I'm upset or angry, I won't go out on the motorbike because that's just stupid, but I might go to the gym and take the stress out in the gym. Physical exercise is something I recommend one hundred per cent because it just increases the endorphins, and it really does make a difference. I don't know how I would be now without the gym, because going to the gym has been a massive thing for me.

For all those going through similar struggles with their mental health, I'd say seek help, don't be scared to talk to somebody and don't be put off by the potential stigma. You're not the only person. There are millions of other people struggling just the same, and the best, the only way to deal with it is to just try and seek some help, however that may be for you – counselling, medication or whatever it is, just don't be afraid to ask for a bit of help. I genuinely hope that my and other people's stories help others, because everybody's story is different. Mine might not seem as bad as someone else's, but everybody's been through a different journey, and I just hope that my story, along with others, will help people.

REFLECTIONS

REFLECTIONS

REFLECTIONS

EIGHT

BEREAVEMENT: MIKE

I'm thirty-six-years-old and yet some days I feel forty-six. I've been a physio for the last fifteen years.

My awareness of my mental health has really come into play since losing my mum in 2015 to breast cancer. Mum was sick for ten years with a diagnosis, and she was in remission for a couple of years, but it was pretty much a ten-year battle with cancer.

It was only really a couple of years, maybe eighteen months, after losing my mum that I acknowledged I was struggling with the bereavement and more generally with mental health.

People talk about a mental health diagnosis in the context of the duration and severity of symptoms and/or signs and symptoms. Mine were persisting probably a lot longer beyond the bereavement to be associated with the bereavement. I started to struggle with everything in my life at that point, and it was a catalyst for hitting rock bottom, which is a cliché phrase, but I think I'd bottomed out.

It's been a journey since losing my mum, with ups and downs, to a point where I'm now in a period of stability with it. After the bereavement I was prompted to seek help and be more open and understanding of my own fundamental health and how best to manage it – the idea of really talking openly about it across the board and similarly wrestling with the fact that it's okay to have days where things aren't quite so bad. I think everybody would love to have days where everything's great, wouldn't they? But that's not the reality for most people, so I still wrestle with that.

When I found out my mum had breast cancer I was only seventeen, so I was quite young, and I remember the day that I found out. My cousin and I were very close, and I went round to him and just broke down to him while he was working. He put his arms around me and hugged me. In hindsight, he was a more outwardly emotional person than I was. I don't even know if I broke down with my family when Mum sat us down to tell us.

I've never not loved my mum, but I was a typical boy in the sense of being too proud in front of my mates to say, "I love you, Mum", which is kind of ridiculous, isn't it? But my cousin was always the other way. He'd be hugging his mum, telling her "I love you, Mum." And she'd say, "Get off", just messing about with him. They had a slightly different kind of relationship, him and my auntie. That's my only recollection, if I'm honest, of any kind of interactions of support that I remember.

Maybe it's a weird age where you may be ignorant of the magnitude and don't quite understand it, but I guess deep down I knew; obviously, I knew it wasn't good. There was a similar pattern to how we dealt with the whole thing over the course of that ten years, where mum would feed my brother and me bits of information and updates, keeping us in the loop. Maybe we didn't know the real ins and outs, the nitty-gritty of stuff that mum and dad did. I think they shielded us from that to some extent.

Having a brief conversation with a chemistry teacher who was feared by everybody, including me, and being on the wrong end of a couple of his tellings off, made it clear the school had been made aware of Mum's situation before I knew, because they anticipated that I may be coming in the next day in a shit state.

The day after my mum told us what was happening, my dad

phoned me during the chemistry class. I looked at my phone and my chemistry teacher looked at me and he just nodded as if to say, "I know. Off you go." It wasn't even a conversation; it was just that knowing, and at that point I remember thinking, people are clearly aware of this. It's weird those things that you pick up on. I've got no real recollection of anybody sitting me down from the school, although I had a sociology teacher who would always ask how Mum was. She would always try and make sure that I was okay, and I think I acted out in that class, which is weird because she was probably the most supportive teacher I remember. I had to re-sit an exam that I didn't really want to re-sit, to be honest; it was to try and get a better grade, but I just walked out of the exam. I started to get a bit more flippant around that time, so I'm surprised I managed to get through school really, in the way that I did, but I wasn't far off finishing when I got the news.

I don't remember a follow-up conversation with my cousin. There will have been, because we were quite close at the time, but it was more about going for beers, that kind of support, without being a sitting down and "let's talk about this."

Once I was in physio I felt an expectation that I would understand a little bit more from a medical point of view, so I had a conversation with my parents to say that I found that quite difficult. I think from then on they closed off a little bit, protected me even more, which then fed me with a little bit of guilt that I wasn't as supportive, in a way. I felt an element of guilt which is still there.

Over the course of that ten years, we dealt with it with humour, really, and Mum had a few hospital admissions. There would be a running joke that I'd be there making her get out of bed. There's a great photograph of me leading my mum on a walk around her room, and then she's in the background of this picture and not best pleased with me, holding up two fingers telling us to "piss off". That's a really cherished photo, and that's how we dealt with it. Our parents tried hard not to burden us, but we had a level of understanding that we knew, especially after the second diagnosis, that ultimately we were on borrowed time, and we tried our best to make the most of that.

We were very fortunate that Mum was in reasonable physical capacity. I wouldn't say health, but she had reasonable physical capacity up until the last two weeks of her life. And then we were very fortunate that mum had real close friends who were in the caring profession who cared for her the last couple of weeks of her life.

I don't know if I would've been able to do that. There might have been a point where I'd have had to, but I never really had to find that out, which I am grateful for. We were lucky that Mum got to be at home when she died, and we managed to have all the family around us. This is one of the most haunting kinds of memory of the whole thing and something that I really have to actively work to push to one side because it can trigger me at any given moment.

Everybody talks about wanting to be there with loved ones when they die, and, given the choice, I would want to be there. But still, sitting and watching somebody you know and love so dearly die in front of you is beyond difficult. You wouldn't want that person to be on their own, but sometimes there's a lot to be said for people dying peacefully in their sleep.

Off the back of that, me, my dad, and my brother had the funeral about two or three weeks later. I've haven't got any real distinct memories of the time in between, but I do remember periods of time where we'd just wander into town, and we did normal life. We went shopping and had lots of people coming round. There were periods of time it was just me, my dad, and my brother in the house, and it just felt a bit empty, like there was a void.

On the day of the funeral, we played some sad songs, as you do, had some remembrance moments, and then she was taken out of the church to some T Rex music to bring some light to it all.

There was a numbness to that day and I don't really remember it very much, to be honest. One of the more noticeable things is that you can't really describe that period to anybody unless they've been in it and lived it. I don't think there is a way of understanding it.

Everybody gets on with their life and just carries on because life doesn't stop for anybody else. I was lucky to have friends who were supportive and around, but sometimes they just had to leave me be and let me get on with the process of bereavement. There was a period where me, my dad, and my brother checked in with each other, and then there's no distinct point when we stopped and went to a normal level of communication.

We were all probably struggling in our own way. We all acknowledged that everybody would be and that we were, but I don't think we necessarily had any outward kind of conversation about it. I tried to get my dad to go and speak to Macmillan Cancer Support, and you just assume that you're doing okay in your own world and try helping others, pushing them towards the services. In hindsight, I was on a slippery slope of struggling over the course of that eighteen months after mum passed away. I found myself not getting joy out of anything. I remember I saw something on Instagram describing depression as this constant rain just raining on you, and that stayed with me. Whatever situation I was in, whatever joy was in that situation was just dampened, and I didn't feel the joy that situation could or should bring. I was becoming more erratic with emotions and being triggered for no apparent reason. I was in this downward spiral, to the point where I can't even really remember the specifics of anything. Then somebody said something that triggered me and made me realise I needed to go and see somebody or be referred to somebody. I self-referred into NHS services. But I don't think I found that particularly helpful. I maybe had two or three sessions with a counsellor.

There were two take-homes for me; one where I was told to drink milk because it made me feel close to my mum, which, maybe there's some science behind it, I don't know. I just remember thinking, 'Is that it? Is that your advice for this situation?' It was because I was not sleeping at night and having panic attacks, but I don't think it helped, to be honest.

The second piece of life advice I remember was that I was that the counsellor said that I was chasing a normal that no longer existed. At the time I was decorating my house, trying to change my job, and my relationship at the time came to an end. I was constantly trying to get back to normal or finding there was a constant reason why I wasn't feeling normal. The reality is that I was trying to get back to a normal that wasn't there anymore. In effect, I was throwing the baby out with the bathwater by changing everything.

Having had counselling since, I'm in a much better place than I was when I had counselling before, and I am more understanding of my own emotions. I had a really good conversation with the counsellor about various sorts of triggers, and it was to do with a previous breakup, which I think triggered some of those emotions of loss that I hadn't experienced since my mum. There's no real similarity between a breakup and bereavement, but there is a sense of loss, that something's been lost, and I think that was the first time I'd felt a sense of loss since losing Mum, so I was close to uncovering some of those previous feelings.

My reintroduction to counselling was far more positive, as it was far more conversational, with a back-and-forth, rather than feeling I was being coached, I guess. It was also with a female counsellor this time, rather than a male one. Maybe there was something maternalistic that put me more at ease.

Maybe it's a male thing. And does that reflect in my life now? I'd say, yeah. The people that I go to for support, for the conversational support, tend to be the girls that I'm friends with. That's not to say that my guy friends are not supportive. The level of support I get from the guys is a bit different in the sense that we go for beers, or get together to train, or go and walk, or keep busy and active. And that's okay. For me, I think it's a bit undervalued, in that I don't think that you always have to have a full kind of "How are you feeling?" conversation, because sometimes people intuitively know that you're not okay and just the fact that you can say, "Come on, we're gonna go for a beer," or go for a walk, just so we can be together and know we will chat about whatever it may be, and if that branches off into "How are you feeling?", great. Let's not undervalue the power of just being in proximity and being with somebody and just feeling their company. It's that bond, you know, "your vibe is your tribe" kind of thing.

As for my panic attacks, there were more than a few over the years, and I still get them now if I'm really stressed or tired, or if I haven't trained. The first major one was when we went away for a holiday to Gibraltar, which is where my brother and I had been to surprise our parents at one of the final stops on one of their cruises.

My brother and I flew over for literally thirty-six hours to meet them off the boat, and we snuck up on them – there's a great video of it.

After Mum died, my dad, brother, and I went back over to visit some family friends for a few days. It must have been within the first year or so of Mum dying.

When we were there, we stayed with our friends in their basement. We went out for food to a place called Mihas for Argentinian steak, and it was amazing. This was in 2016 and it was around about the time that a Formula One driver had their house broken into after someone pumped gas into their house and basically knocked them out, sent them to sleep and then broke in. I don't know why that stays with me, but the first time I had one of these panic attacks, it happened in our friend's basement. It was pitch black, which made me feel like I was suffocating. I was in this real panic state of screaming, to the dismay of my brother, who was in the same room as me, in this other single bed. He was obviously in a blind panic and we were both running around, bumping into each other and into furniture because it was pitch black, there was no light whatsoever. Then everybody upstairs heard what was going on and the lights started coming on and they started asking, "What the hell is going on?" I reassured them with "I'm okay, I'm all right." But everyone else was not okay.

In hindsight, the first one I ever had was before Mum died. That was a very minor event in that I'd get up and race to the window, searching behind the radiator for some unknown reason, and my brother was again in the same room asking, "What the hell is happening?", then I'd settle down. The one in Spain was the first major one, and I've never had any major one again after that, but they became a little bit more regular in terms of not sleeping well, and that's where the conversation with the counsellor came in, to some extent. Waking every night in cold sweats and tears, with the feeling of being suffocated. Like I said, it still happens now when I'm stressed, have a lot on my plate, or I'm worried about something or not sure what's going to happen with something in my life. They are far less extreme, but still have that common suffocating sensation. I take this as a warning sign now that I need to train, to look after myself a little bit better.

Having these mental health issues clearly affects your family. My dad and I go through ups and downs generally anyway. My relationship with my dad goes through good patches and bad patches, and that's partly to do with him wanting to be more involved, because he recognises when I'm not in a good place, or when I'm not content, that kind of thing. He wants to be able to support me, but for whatever reason I don't feel like I have that relationship with him, and the capacity to have those conversations with him. I don't think that is a "him" thing, it's more of a "me" thing. My brother and I are very, very close, and it's not quite subconscious, but it's there and he knows. For example, during my last breakup, I didn't have a conversation with either of them to say I'd broken up with my partner, it was just that that person disappeared and wasn't spoken about. I don't really know why that is; again, maybe it's just a man thing, maybe I don't want to burden them, maybe I don't want to put it on them. That's not to say that I feel unsupported by them in any way, far from it. My preference for where I get that type of support sits elsewhere within my friendship groups, and that proximity, because they're a lot closer by.

My friends have seen me more on those really bad days, just because of them being close by. One friend in particular, Sarah, lived with me for a period of a year after Mum died. She saw warts and all in that year. It's quite hard, really, in the sense that you don't want to become the person in the group that's the supported "victim", for want of a better word – the one who's constantly needing levels of support. I'm conscious of that and want to be an active contributor and a supportive person as well. You want it to be a two-way relationship, to have that balance. Am I the more supported? Maybe. And after you become conscious of that dynamic, you don't want to be the burden in the group. Sometimes that's the feeling when you are amongst this kind of stuff because you know they have their stuff going on as well. This is the kind of stigma that we perceive there to be, a self-perceived one in many cases.

I remember writing something a few years ago in Mental Health Awareness Week, outlining all of this stuff in this piece of writing, and I remember the fear of putting it out there, not knowing if it was the right thing to do; but I did it and I would never retract it. I got so many different messages from people saying, "Thank you for writing this", and some of the conversations were just incredible off the back of it, from people you just don't suspect, who come to you and tell you they find it difficult to speak to people about it.

Even in sharing this kind of stuff, you have that feeling of 'Am I doing this for attention, or are people going to *think* that I'm doing this for attention?' I don't think that's the case for me. There's a perception of me sometimes – I'm 6'2", nearly 100 kilos, I'm a big burly man – and I share these aspects of mental health because I want to try and break down those barriers and stigmas, such as men crying. I cry, probably once a week. I find some stuff heartbreaking, and I'm comfortable with the fact that I cry. I was at a wedding a couple of weeks ago and the groom was talking about losing his dad, and we were sat at a horseshoe shaped table, and I was sat looking directly at the bride listening to this speech, and I was gone. I was an absolute mess. And she was looking at me and asking me, "Are you okay?" I told her, "I'm fine, but not really." And then she told me afterwards, "I had no idea you'd be a crier." It's just that perception, and for me that's why I try to be fairly open and outward about this kind of stuff. I'm not always okay, and sometimes you need to get that support from friends. When I'm not okay, I know I can go to just be around people, go for a beer or a cup of tea and not feel like I need to be "Here's all my problems"; just that presence of being around people is sometimes enough.

Whenever I speak to somebody who has had a bereavement, the first thing I tell them is, "I understand that there's no way that you can articulate how you're feeling", and in the early stages of bereavement, it's not something that you can describe to somebody. If somebody literally said, "How are you feeling?" or "What are you feeling?" I don't think you could tell others, and if you could in any way try and articulate it, that person couldn't feel it. I know from my point of view that things will get better with time. It's a massive cliché, but time does heal.

My relationship with everything around the bereavement, especially the anniversary of Mum passing, has changed as it is evolving over time. You make more peace with it. The key thing for me was that there was definitely a conscious decision to talk to people about it and knowing when to be around and not be around people. Sometimes friends had to drag me to the gym, or drag me out of the house, making sure I was doing stuff and keeping me busy. Then that flips and you take a little bit of onus on yourself to remind yourself, "I need to do more. I need to get involved with certain things and speak to people about this kind of stuff."

Sometimes that wasn't through choice, such as when Sarah was living with me. Sometimes I'd be sat on the sofa just as she'd come home, and I would be a mess. Sometimes you have no choice but to talk about it. You also have to make an active decision to speak to somebody, try and articulate to some extent what your struggles are and that things aren't okay. It doesn't have to be an elaborate kind of articulation of how you're feeling, just that things are not okay. And that person generally will have some suggestion about how and where to get the best type of support or work with you to explore what those next steps are.

REFLECTIONS

REFLECTIONS

REFLECTIONS

NINE

FEAR: RICHARD

I'm forty years young and head of operations for a health care company. We develop medical devices. Prior to that, I was in the food industry for about fifteen years. My career started out in the building trade as I took over the family business. I've been in quite a few demanding industries, and I found my feet in manufacturing.

For as long as I can remember, I've always tended to overprocess or overthink things. I think it's the best description that I can give. From an incredibly early age I had tendencies to worry about certain circumstances, such as parents leaving and going to work. I remember circumstances where we'd be in a family environment and I would worry. I was physically sick at one point, and that was my sister's sixteenth birthday. I would have been six, as she's ten years older than me.

Being so young, I had no explanation of the causes or the internalisation of "What's going on? What's happening?" because I'm the type of person who needs to know answers. I must have answers; otherwise, I can't function. It's one of those traits that can be great, but it's also a trait that's quite destructive at the same time.

I can remember episodes of feeling uncomfortable to the point where I was physically sick, and looking back now, was it anxiety? Was it mental health issues? I absolutely one hundred per cent feel that it was, although it wasn't diagnosed that early on, and I think mental health in the late 1980s and early 1990s really wasn't a curriculum. It wasn't taught, it wasn't well known. People had mental health issues but wouldn't have necessarily been diagnosed with anything – not like it is today.

Being that young, and I'm talking less than ten, at that age there was no doctor's visit. My parents knew that in certain circumstances I would feel physically sick or *be* physically sick, and I can remember my mum used to purposely take me into social situations. Was it social anxiety I was experiencing? Was it a generalised anxiety? Who knows? A bit of both, I would say. And that was all spawned from that very first event.

Mum used to take me into cafes where it was busy, and there was the smell of food and whatever other sensory things that were going off. She used to sit me down and bribe me with a sausage roll and a hot chocolate, which I remember to this day. She used to take me into a cafe in Buxton and sit me down, and I'd nervously sit there and drink hot chocolate with a flake and a bit of cream, and through that persistence of what she did, it got me to a point where I would go into busy locations, and I became more socially active.

Now there were a few, and again, interestingly, thinking back, there were probably a few circumstances that would have brought about uncomfortable situations in social environments. When I was young, we lived in the middle of the countryside, so we lived out in what we English like to call "the sticks." Social groups were minimal. My social group was my family and school. There was a school bus, and they were the only social interactions I had at that age. Whereas people of my age now, at that time would have had friendship groups, play dates, and a lot more interaction.

From a community and society perspective, I can clutch at straws and try to pinpoint things, but it isn't going to do me any good. What I do know is that I felt what I felt, I did what I did physically, and my parents at that time were very proactive in getting me back into social situations, which was great.

Jumping forward into my teens, there were episodes when I felt anxious. I can remember specifically being on the couch one evening and watching *EastEnders*. And I stood up and went, "Oh God, my heart's racing." There was no warning of this. It was just literally as I was lying on the sofa watching *EastEnders* and suddenly this wave of emptiness came across me. I was around the age of thirteen or fourteen at this point. And at that age, it was scary.

I can remember going to my mum in the kitchen; it was dark outside and I said to my mum, "I'm not right, Mum." I told her I had this nervous energy, enough nervous energy to run a marathon. I felt like that was what I needed to do. Although I was always very conscious about my heart and thinking, "God, it's beating out." It was quite alarming and concerning in terms of symptoms; it was a fast heart rate, palpitations. It was sweating, cold sweat, a heightened sense of my senses. Sometimes when I was having anxiety attacks, my vision went perfect, my hearing, my taste. Everything that was a primary sense was really exaggerated and crystal clear. A state of euphoric kind of concentration. Very strange, as that episode came and went. That and a few other episodes would last a few days, or even a few weeks.

As I got older certain relationships with my girlfriends impacted me. As it's an emotional time, you can put it down to being a teenager with hormones raging, or you're reacting and learning to become an adult. There's a lot of social pressure in terms of what you want to do, should you go to university or not. "We should do this." "She shouldn't do that." And I was never really the type of person to just conform. I always wanted to do my own thing. I was extremely ambitious, very driven in terms of my career. Having this anxiety in certain elements of my life was impactful, but as a sufferer, it was certainly something that I didn't know how to control.

A few years after I had started driving, I witnessed a horrific road traffic collision involving a pedestrian, and the impact, unfortunately, killed the victim involved. It was horrific and was very much like a scene out of a hospital drama such as *Casualty*. That and a bit more, because you've got your other senses, you've got the smells and the sounds that you don't really get when you're watching a programme, and to this day, I can still smell that specific smell. Visually, it wasn't pleasant, especially as it was a catastrophic accident. There wasn't a straight bone in that gentleman's body, and he was more than likely killed on impact because of the speed at which the car was travelling. Being the first on the scene, there was no one else around. It was dark, and I would have been in my early twenties. The emergency services took quite some time to get there because it was in the remote area of the Hope Valley in Derbyshire. I can remember talking to the first police officer who arrived on the scene. He was polite and asked, "Are you okay? Was there anyone else involved?"

The person who had hit the pedestrian had stopped and turned the car around, and he was not in a good way with his state of mind. The police officer wandered off, and I can remember thinking to myself, 'Oh, you know the victim's over there, he's on the floor, we've covered him up, aren't you going to go and check just to make sure I've got things right?' But he just wandered off, which I believe was his way of saying, "This is too much." He'd hit his limit, and I appreciate that now, but at the time I was like, "Well, you're the professional here!"

The traffic officer arrived, then the fire brigade, and then the ambulance. The traffic officer was almost joking about the situation, and I couldn't believe he was joking about this. I was angry with him because I was thinking, 'You've got a dead man on the floor and you're making a joke out of it!?' It's only in later life that I've realised it was his way of processing what was in front of him, it was his way of being able to cope with what I'm sure is a very high-pressure job. The emergency services deal with some absolutely horrific incidents, and to me it was a one-off incident. Not everyone witnesses that in their lifetime, and I hope no one else does. But to me that was the only thing that mattered. Whereas, you know, if you think about a police officer or emergency services, they deal with these things all the time and they have their own coping mechanisms.

Part of the process of understanding the situation and not being angry at that situation is something I've only realised in later life. For me now, that incident of me being the witness was quite a journey. And when I say a journey, I mean a journey of understanding: "Who am I?" "What do I believe in?" "Is there a God?" "What about my faith?"

I was raised as a Christian. I went to Christian school and started to question an awful lot about life. I don't want to make this religious, but I went into a period of quite deep overthinking and overprocessing.

The inquest for the accident, which happened in September 2006, took place around January 2007. Thinking I was fine up until that point, but not recognising a lot of triggers, I had become a self-employed builder with a busy schedule. When the coroner's letter landed on the doorstep, I remember thinking, "God, this is an inconvenience. I'm so busy I can't afford the time off. I'm not going to get paid for this," but on the day of the inquest, I jumped in my Land Rover Discovery thinking, "God, I've just got to get there, get it done, and get back." As I set off I was feeling this elevated level of pressure. There were a lot of things going off in my head, and I can remember looking at the radio move around the vehicle. I kid you not. I've never had any hallucinations. I've had a drink or two in my time and the room's been spinning, but I've never witnessed anything like that in my life: the radio just going around the windscreen. I instantly had a hit of adrenaline and high, high anxiety, and it felt like my soul had dropped out of me. I felt empty and to the point where I don't know how I got to the coroner's court. I really don't. I sat in the courtroom and listened for what felt like days. I was asked to give my statement and then suffered two years of what I now know was PTSD.

Immediately after the coroner's inquest it was a downward spiral quite quickly. It was everything that you can imagine: high anxiety, weight loss, being immobile when it came to any kind of physical activity. I dropped a couple of stone in weight, and I wasn't a big guy anyway, so two stone is quite precious. Every symptom that you can imagine from constant anxiety attacks, including a lack of sleep, which I think is one of my biggest enemies and my Achilles heel right now.

Going to the doctors at my worst was an almost daily occurrence, and they were trying to prescribe me antidepressants at one point to shut me up and turn me away, which I think was their tactic. In the early 2000s, was mental health really spoken about? No.

Due to the fact I was self-employed, I was losing money as well and spent a lot of money on alternative therapies. At my worst, I ended up in A&E (Accident and Emergency) and it was a journey that I'll always remember. I was with my father, and we were out on a job quite late in the day. I think he was fed up with me being in the house and not really motivated to do anything. He'd said, "Come on, let's go!" So we set off. We were fitting a kitchen at the time, and we were a few miles down the road when this wave of tingly sensations, akin to pins and needles, started in my toes. I thought to myself, 'Oh, that's strange', and slowly but surely it started to work its way into my foot, into my ankles, and then up my calf, into my legs, into my knees, and then my fingers started to tingle as well. That moved across my arms, into my forearm, into my bicep and then into my chest. And it got to the top of my torso and into my groin area; and I turned to my dad and said, "You know I love you, Dad, and I think I'm dying. I think I'm dying."

He looked at me and asked, "What do you mean?" I told him, "I've got this feeling, and I can't describe it." It was horrific.

He responded with, "Right, OK, well, we'll get you to hospital." And I remember to this day, I turned to him and said, "I love you."

We got to A&E, and he pushed me out of the car because there was typically nowhere to park, and he wasn't willing to just drive around the car park waiting for a parking space. I remember I opened the door of A&E and I literally fell onto the floor, and a triage nurse came over with the receptionist and put me in a wheelchair, and she asked, "What's the matter?" So I told her, "I'm dying."

Looking back now, I can laugh and think, 'Wow, that was a pretty dark place, you know, a pretty bad place that you were in, Richard!'

Was I depressed? I would say so, yes. I'd been suffering for such a long time with no real let-out, with no real avenue to express feelings or emotions. Were relationships hindered and tainted? Absolutely. I lost a lot of friends, lost a girlfriend, and that was tough.

The process of being in A&E was the starting point of my recovery, and it started with a nurse who came to me and told me, "You know, you're OK. You're fine, and you need to pull yourself together." These were her exact words. We look at that now and think, 'God, what was she saying? What was she thinking? How can you say that to someone who is suffering?' and I did take it that way. I really did. And I absolutely felt the anger, bitterness and everything else along those lines. But I'm also the type of person that looks at those sorts of situations and says, "Thank you. I thank you for making that comment because you pissed me off in that moment of truth." She shouldn't have said that, not professionally, absolutely not; but I used that as fuel to put me on a trajectory of recovery.

I didn't know it at the time, and it took many, many years to look back and think that was the absolute rock-bottom that I hit. That turned me around.

What was the recovery?

The recovery was learning about what was going on. It was about finding alternative methods of coping, and I always describe it as a little toolbox. You carry this toolbox throughout your whole life. And at the start it's quite empty. You've got the fight-and-flight response and that's all you've got.

From an early age, we can run or we can fight, and that's all we've got. As we get older, we learn to cope with certain situations.

There are all sorts of big life events that happen. Bereavement, relationships, marriage, births; these are all things that get put into our toolbox for us to learn. We learn the ways to deal with things, and it's no different with anxiety. We learn to cope.

Will it always be there?

"I don't know" is the answer, but if it does arrive back, then I've now got the right tools and I've got the right friends and support group that will get me through it. Understanding what the triggers are is a huge thing for me in my period of life now. I know that if I don't eat well, if I don't sleep, if I have a period of prolonged stress – whether that's physical stress, such as if I go to the gym too much, or the mental stress of work and a home life of having two young children at home – then I can get triggered.

It's been a very interesting process. I'm going to call it a process of learning about who I am, what actually makes me tick, of not falling into that kind of societal pressure of "You must do this, you must be married and have children, go to university, get this, earn this amount of money, et cetera, et cetera. I've been truly fortunate in that I've found several people who have helped me in ways that they don't even understand. But finding my feet in learning about myself, about depression and anxiety, can happen so quickly and yet so silently.

And I suppose that's the thing for me; I know the things that keep me on the straight and narrow. I don't want to sound too dramatic, but it is a constant, it's like staying fit. You know if you're going to eat at McDonald's every day, at some point you're going to put on a few pounds. Just like if I don't practise meditation, or do yoga, or maybe if I don't sleep well for a week, or if I'm not eating the right foods for a week, I know I'm going to feel pretty rough. I'm going to feel a little bit detached, a little bit disjointed. I am not going to have the clarity to think normally if I don't do the healthier things.

It's these life choices that we can make, and they are absolutely in our hands to move us forward into a better place.

Is it fear that keeps us in that cycle? It is to a certain extent, and I appreciate that everyone's story is different, but I had a real fear of dying, of having a heart attack or heart failure. I had a desire to find a way that I could survive, and I could live normally.

And I always go back to that nurse because everyone I talked to about the nurse telling me "Pull yourself together" is in absolute disbelief: "What the hell!? How could she have said that to you?" But I used that in a unique way, and I think about it differently. I used it as a battery and a cell of energy to push me in a different direction.

The mental health journey did affect my relationships with friends and family, and in a positive way, because we've always been quite close, and my openness has certainly helped my brother, as he has had his time as well. From a family unit point of view, it's helped us to be more open and talk about mental health. I think my dad has always struggled to conceptualise and understand truly what it is, because my dad is so laid back he's horizontal! I often joke with him, "Where the hell did I get this from!? Who's responsible for this chromosome!? Who can I hang this one on?" As a family, it made us closer, although certain members of the family didn't understand it.

In terms of social peer groups, because I'm so open, I found out who my loyal friends were. Some didn't really understand, whereas others really helped. Some of them were like the nurse and said pull yourself together, and others were a lot more understanding, and I found some amazing friends through that process and had a bit of a clear-out. We all have social media of one description, shape or size these days. How many friends of those hundreds of people do you speak to? And I think through this process I got down to four or five that that really understood, and that was quite nice actually. That was nice.

In terms of relationships, in terms of intimate relationships with girlfriends, one hundred per cent it did impact the relationships. I would say my mental health also impacted my financial capability to make decisions, properly informed decisions. Not going into it too much, but say you have some credit, for example, and you're in a state of mind where you're thinking, 'Well, I could die tomorrow' or 'I feel like crap, I'll go and buy a luxury item, such as a hot tub' because you haven't got to pay for it. I've been there and suffered huge consequences of then having to pay the bloody thing back with a silly amount of interest. Cars were a passion for me, so I spent a ridiculous amount on cars and then struggled financially to pay the money back. I've made some terrible decisions in terms of my finances because of this state of mind.

Absolutely, mental health impacts the whole of your life. It's not just one area, it has so many knock-on effects and domino effects on all areas of your life.

In terms of professional support, I sought help with my journey in the first instance with my GP at the local doctor's surgery. I've had CBT (cognitive behavioural therapy) and had several talk therapists as well, which I found quite useful as I found some tools in there that helped me be able to cope with things. I think on my journey it's been quite interesting for me personally because I suffered with anxiety from such a young age. I got to a certain point in my life where I thought, 'You know what, I'm on top of this, these symptoms. I'm fine, I can manage it with the tools that I've got.'

And then, lo and behold, because our brain is so clever, it changes the way it catches you out. So it changed the symptoms, and I was like, "Oh God, this is something different. It is definitely a brain tumour, it's definitely a heart issue." And then I had to learn over again how to cope with that. It may have meant a different kind of clinician. It may have meant a different therapy. It may have meant diverse ways of coping. In my latter stages I've tried acupuncture and regressive therapy (which really didn't work and never has worked for me personally, and I steer clear of that sort of thing now).

What I found worked was massage, which was really beneficial for me personally. I also found meditation and yoga to be positive. Everyone is different, and it's a trial-and-error scenario. You must go and try a few things, see what feels comfortable and fits, and then you can digest it accordingly.

True professional help was limited due to long waiting lists, even back then in the early 2000s. In 2010, I had to wait twelve weeks to see a CBT therapist, which is three months of coping on your own before you even get to share your story. . I can remember filling out forms at work, thinking, 'Should I tick that box? Should I let them know that?' There has been that issue, and now I believe we should absolutely tick the box and share our story, because that is who we are. But back then, I avoided sharing thoughts because I thought I would be viewed differently, and maybe I would have been. Perhaps if I'd ticked those boxes it would have been different. I've never been held back and victimised for my mental health, so I think I've been lucky in that sense.

There's an open environment in the company I work for now, which is fantastic. We do so much with mind and mental health, and being open and honest, and having sessions where people can talk openly. We do so much around the menopause and the way women struggle in that period of their life too, as well as a lot for charity.

It is a vastly different world right now in terms of the commercial world; some companies are particularly good at dealing with mental health, and others are not. We have just sent three people on a mental health first aid training course, of which I'm a huge advocate, for obvious reasons.

I suppose a lot of my drive is to try and help people in terms of the stigma in the world right now, and sadly, I know at least four or five people who have committed suicide in the last two years.

Recently I read on LinkedIn about a son of a colleague who had killed himself. This was a young lad in his twenties who had a first-class honours degree and so much potential, and yet because there's this stigma in society that ignites the voice in your head and telling you, "I can't suffer with that! Why should I have to go and speak to someone?" we end up suffering alone as this young lad did.

Our purpose must be to offer olive branches and be able to recognise and contact people in their darkest moments.

Keeping the faith when we are in that darkness, keeping one eye on the "What if?" of when you're in *that* place, "What if there is very little light at the end of the tunnel?" when there's very little enjoyment in life, or there's very little means of being joyful yourself, being able to put on a fake smile or a fake laugh can make all the difference.

You may attend parties where everyone else seems to be having fun, and you look around the room and see people enjoying themselves and you almost feel guilty for not being able to enjoy that yourself.

Through everything that I've experienced, and from talking to other people, what differentiates me or makes me different to others is that I always tried to say to myself, "I will find a way of coping" or "There will be another tool that will arrive unexpectedly", and at some point, there will be another friend who offers a piece of advice that will carry you through.

There'll be a nurse that tells you to pull yourself together, and whether that's right or wrong, you will find certain elements of fuel to keep one eye on that horizon; and I think what's really important is that just a small shimmer and glimmer of hope will actually carry you through. Don't underestimate how resilient you are. We talk about so many things in society that are wrong, but we don't talk about the things that are great. We've survived on this planet for millions of years. We've gone through millions of different traumatic circumstances, and as a human race we have survived, and that's exactly what someone in this situation will do.

REFLECTIONS

REFLECTIONS

TEN

BULLYING: ROB

This event happened in my past. I was lucky that I had something that, post-COVID, a lot of people have now, which is a strong support network.

I was and still am lucky that in various situations my life is fine, and I've moved on. But what horrifies me is that the same history is repeating itself again and again.

I'm in a sports group, and I was speaking to one of my friends a few weeks ago, just a casual conversation over drinks about work, and I said, "How's work going?"

And the answer was, "Oh, terrible bosses." I made a throwaway comment: "Yeah, I had one years ago. It was absolutely horrible. This female boss made my life miserable, whether she intended to or not, through bullying at work."

Like I said, a throwaway comment. And interestingly, this friend of mine looked at me with wide eyes and said, "Really? How do you mean?" So I told him a little bit more and he replied with, "That's … I'm actually having the same situation at the moment." I opened up more about how it affected me and what happened.

Obviously, he's a friend of mine. I'm in contact with him almost daily, and the thing here is, because of the stigma, it's not clinical, it's not scientific.

I don't send him a message saying, "How are you feeling?" It's more, "You all right, mate? How's things? What you up to?" and we both read between the lines.

He called me up about ten days ago. Men have a tendency to want to find answers to things, but he just needed to talk *at* me and unload, and we had a fifteen- or twenty-minute conversation. I said about three sentences. It was just that the pressure was weighing on him so much that he needed to get that off his chest, and at the end of it he said, "Thanks for listening. I really needed that. I'll see you around." And that was it.

It horrifies me because, as I said, history is repeating itself.

My personal story happened when I had finished university and started my first job in the city. To gain this this role, I'd gone through quite a detailed process of being interviewed and had about five interviews I'd created example projects for. The lady who would be my direct manager had chosen to put me through the first two phases. She'd determined that my projects were of suitable calibre. I was then interviewed by her again, and I think the final two were with her and a senior director who was male.

We're encouraged to go out and show confidence, and that sometimes means that our confidence can be misconstrued, particularly if we don't understand how to convey confidence. It can be misconstrued as aggression. It can also be misconstrued as being pushy. Passive confidence, I think, is quite a challenging thing to demonstrate so that it doesn't offend or worry people.

Starting this new job was a female junior at the same level as me. We were both in this team as a team of two, both of us reporting to this female manager, and we were both new starts on the same day.

The female new start is a close friend of mine. I introduced her to another friend of mine, and they got engaged and married.

It was interesting how we were meant to be given the same training, but certain aspects were missing in my training, as I discovered retrospectively. I did my best to develop in this job, working at it, but things didn't go well for me because if I hadn't done something in the right time frame or if a certain file hadn't been submitted, on time or at all, problems started escalating. I would ask myself, "Why can't I get this? Because this is the field I've chosen. This is what I understand. This is what I know. My grades were good. They said the project I'd submitted was great. They gave me the job. I have trained with my colleague, and she and I should be able to get this right, so I don't know why I keep getting things wrong." So first you start with self-doubt, because you don't question an outside source to begin with. First you start to shift. *What am I doing wrong?* Then it's *I'm obviously not capable* or *I'm not intelligent* or *I'm not good enough.*

Thankfully, I'm now in a happy, stable situation with relationships, et cetera, so I can look back with hindsight, and those three interpretations (I'm not capable, I'm not intelligent, I'm not good enough) start to snowball. Normally you might be able to pigeonhole work, and then you've got your social life, sports or whatever, but suddenly those three statements start spiralling into other areas of your life. So, "No, I'm not good enough for that competition", etc.

The little voice in your head starts; normally that little voice is quiet, but with those three statements hanging over you, every single day, Monday to Friday, you're having it reaffirmed. *"You're the problem. Others are doing fine. They're doing the same thing. You're the issue. You're the problem."* And that voice gets louder and louder and then it starts saying, *"No, actually, I can't take that shot. I'm not capable. I'm not going to do it because I'm not good enough"*, and like a mushroom, it grows and grows.

To this day, I remember two things – well, multiple things – which happened over a period of about a year and a half. Part of my job was negotiations, particularly telephone negotiations, so we're going back to when I first entered the world of work here, when Zoom and all that sort of stuff didn't exist. We worked internationally, so it's very much about how you communicate over the phone. And there are two things that stand out in my memory. One was that picking up the phone, I realised I was so depressed that I answered the phone,

"Hello. Yes," and I was on the verge of tears because the depression had got to such a level.

I got told off for answering the phone in an incorrect fashion that would affect the business. The irony is that the situation that had been created in my mind had spiralled to such a point that then it was *actually* affecting my work. The concept that my work was being affected had grown in my own head and was being reaffirmed because I was being told on a daily basis by my female boss, verbatim words: "You're useless," "Why don't you know this?" And you think, "Well, I'm sure I haven't been told this."

But you don't dare question it for fear that it's politically incorrect, that you might offend someone, and you don't dare question that, particularly not your direct senior.

The second thing that always stays with me is the female colleague who came up to me one lunchtime and said, "I don't understand why, when you ask a question about a process or something else, you get shouted at, but when I ask a question, I get an immediate answer or 'I'll answer you as soon as I can'." My colleague told me, "If you need something, message me via MSM Messenger, and I'll ask it." Back then we sat in an open-plan office with desks facing one another in a horseshoe-style formation, and so I would message her, she would ask the question, the female manager would respond to her and I would get the answer.

I raised it with the director, and back then issues of workplace bullying were not as prevalent as they are today and the concept was not understood. There weren't processes, so I was incredibly lucky that he was understanding; but the way he dealt with it was to talk to me and encourage me to work harder. I was already getting in before everyone, leaving after everyone, and double-checking everything, and I just thought, 'yeah, OK', and he said, "If you've got issues, come to me", and so it was only through that process, the support of the senior boss and my colleague, that I managed to go through this for about a year and a bit.

I knew I had hit rock-bottom when the suicidal thoughts were strong and I'd wake up in the morning after a nice deep sleep, the alarm clock would off, and before the alarm had stopped, I'd have that awakening of "yes, I am awake", and tears would roll down my face before I'd got the duvet off, because I was sad to be awake, to be alive, to be going back into that place. And of course, people will say, "Just change. Why did you stick with it? Why, if it was that terrible?" Again, as a young man, you get on that treadmill, and I was in a flat share, I was in a contract, there was rent to pay, there were rates to pay, there were bills to pay; and you not only have the stigma of having gotten your first job and everyone wants you to do well, to walk out and have people asking, "What? Why? Why did you walk out?" If you responded with, "I was being bullied" then you'd be hit with, "What do you mean, being bullied?" Back then it was the concept that bullying was the preserve of the schoolyard. And if you complained about bullying in a workplace, then you would be mocked, and no one would comprehend. Stigma still exists, and sadly, I don't think it's got much better.

I was truly fortunate that I was in a flat share with two guys, and they were slightly older than me, and there was nothing scientific about it whatsoever, but they could clearly see from the way I acted and locked myself away that something was wrong. It wasn't scientific, and I'm sure any expert would be horrified by the way they dealt with it, but what they helped me do was force me to partition, to try and get equilibrium back in my life. If I had to be in that environment five days a week during the working day, then I had to make sure that I was distracted when I wasn't at work, so I wasn't thinking about it.

It's probably wrong and bad, but there was a lot of heavy drinking and a lot of playing the board game Risk. There was a lot of going to parties, and the thoughts that had been affecting my social life and sports teams – "I can't do this" – became "Well, actually, you can. You've been doing this for years. You're good at this sport, so go on."

Even someone you've only lived with for a brief period, when you chat and say, "Oh, yes, I'm a rugby player. We play on Wednesdays," and they say, "I'll come watch," and Wednesday arrives and you're not getting ready, your flatmates say, "Shouldn't you be playing tonight?" They see that you're missing out on those things, and so they actively pushed and encouraged. The other great thing that they did was to take me to a working men's club which they were members of.

The new term, which many people still don't comprehend, is *male safe spaces*. And it's sad that these concepts that are traditional to people my father's age or older, these traditional safe spaces have been eroded. Working men's clubs, drinking pubs where depression gets solved. Personally, in my experience, it doesn't get solved by sitting down in a clinical atmosphere with someone in a lab coat saying, "Why are you depressed? Tell me about your emotions." Men don't like that. What does happen, a bit like the friend that I had, is you get to disclosures as they call them, around about pint four or five over a general conversation, and you don't home in on it. It's like, "Oh dear, are you OK there?" It's touched on, and the conversation moves away, then it comes back again. And that's how we communicate with tough things. We can't go head-on with it. All respect to the ladies, they're much better at dealing with this kind of stuff than we are because we like to go round and round and attack it from different angles and eventually you get there. I was fortunate that I had a male supportive home environment. Supportive being very traditional, you know, "Here have a pint," type thing, but that was almost the important part for me. They weren't asking me about my emotions, they were just trying to give me a plateau, to give me the yin and the yang.

And you know, I didn't bottle everything up. As a young man I spoke to my parents, my family, and said, "This is terrible, I hate it. I don't seem to be able to do anything right." They told me, of course, to stick at it, try it. "You've got bills to pay, so you can't just walk out because the rent is due regardless."

It's my first job straight out of uni. Everybody catches up with each other. "How's it going? Oh yes, I'm doing well. It's kind of, well, you know, I've got to just try and make this work; and you? How's things with you?"

The senior director repeated the same thing from the other side: stick at it, focus. It was over a year before I started having suicidal thoughts. Though, ironically, it wasn't until I got the confidence to confide in him that I couldn't cope, that life should not be like this. I shouldn't wake up and cry because I have to come to work. I'm not saying I should be jumping out of bed and running up the street to get to work, but I should at least be quite pleased to see the people in the office.

As a first job, my first working experience, I have nothing to compare it to, but life shouldn't be like this. I told him, "I'm going to, you know, I can't stand it anymore. I have thought about ending it. Something has to change, and I can't be stuck here." And he said, "Just give me one more month." I kept thinking, 'No! Why? What would that possibly do? I've suffered enough. I know I'm getting ill frequently. I joined this company a fit athlete and my weight's gone up. I'm getting ill. I'm drinking ridiculous amounts.' Although that was actually part of the coping strategy.

But it was insane. The alcoholism was through the roof, and I was living for the weekend. I would come home and have a pint of vodka orange as soon as I got through the door, and I was probably having four a night just to try and create a barrier to stop any thoughts of work either today or what would happen tomorrow, or having to deal with it all. It was just me trying to create a capsule.

Anyway, I trusted him, so I stayed for my sins. We would have our conversations over a packed lunch. We'd walk to the park, just out the office, and I see now that these lunches could have been because I was having this issue with this female manager – who was not answering my questions, was putting me down in front of everyone and saying that my work was bad. Which made my work bad because my mental health deteriorated. The worse it got, the more I lunched with him, and of course that made the situation worse, and it got to the point where one day we went out for lunch and he said, "She's leaving."

Again, for my sins, I wept. I wept with happiness, and he was absolutely aghast. I had to ask him to repeat it a couple of times because of the relief. The irony is that immediately my work shone through, and about three months later I got promoted because, even though she had drilled it into me that I couldn't do it, that I wasn't any good, that I wasn't capable, that the work was rubbish, it turned out that the reason she hired me was because I *was* good at my job. Yet my work and I had been smothered with the equivalent of a fire blanket, and as soon as that blanket was removed the quality of my work was seen, and the results increased. It was then a very happy working environment, and slowly my life got back to normal.

My sport picked up again, and I realised, "Yeah, I am good at this." Then it was a case of, "Well, actually, no, I don't want that pint of vodka because I've got a match and I've got training, so no." If I hadn't had that network of mostly male support, at home, from the male senior just telling me to steer the course, stay at it, I don't think I would have gotten through this.

Fast-forward five years and I had a similar experience at a reunion with university friends. We were in the pub. We hadn't seen each other for a while and there was a broad spectrum of us; there was a teacher, a scientist, one was in sales and one was an accountant. We were four of us standing in the street, just chatting, saying, "yes, things are good", "sport's well", "job's fine", and then we moved on to relationships. One of the chaps told us, "I broke up with *X*" and he didn't come to it immediately, tells us and we all say, "sorry about that," so we went away from the subject. We came back to it, and it was about the third coming-back-to-subject where everyone had talked about their relationships vaguely and "oh, yeah, it's great" when this one chap said that his ex was saying she was pregnant. It had been a messy breakup, and again, it's not scientific in any way, shape or form, but it was really intriguing that of the four of us, three of us had been emotionally blackmailed about a fake pregnancy. And the older one, who'd always been the team leader of our friendship group, said, "Oh, my God, I'm with you. I've been there." This gave us the confidence in sharing. Men are terrible at talking about stuff; it is interesting how we're unbelievably bad at talking and how those things affect us.

There's a stigma about showing any form of openness, any chink in the armour, particularly to a lady. I needed that female colleague; if she hadn't been there asking the questions that I wasn't allowed to ask – those simple work questions, not the tough emotional ones – I wouldn't have been able to keep going in the job.

I was incredibly grateful that I had that balance of camaraderie in an all-male space of the working men's club, playing pool of a weekend and having my flatmates, that environment of older sage advice. I didn't go in, "Oh, woe is me" but it's amazing how in general conversation people tell you about their experiences, particularly older men who seem to like to talk at the bar; some of their stuff wasn't relevant to my situation in any way, shape or form, but it reminded me that, actually, if I stopped the myopic and tunnel-vision thinking, being in this little bubble where everything was bad and I was no good at it – whatever *it* was – and just listened to other people talking about what they were doing, it was actually a reminder that I didn't have that myopia, that it's not all about me and there's a world outside if I just stop and look and chip away at the bricks. It was a great separator which helped departmentalize everything for me, and I'm fairly sure it would have been a different result if I weren't brave, if I hadn't stuck my hand up and confided in the senior person at work.

The working world was a different world for me, and I was naturally scared that I'd be seen as the bad guy; I was the new guy, after all. It wasn't a politically correct thing to say, and I wasn't sure how it'd be taken, so I didn't put my hand up. I didn't ask for help. I said I had a problem in that environment, and the people that supported me were the network around me.

It's scary, and the whole topic of men's mental health is quite of interest to me, having gone through it. I read a statistic that post-pandemic, men have very few male friends, and those safe spaces are gone. It's cheaper to buy drinks in the supermarket and watch Netflix, so pubs are closing at a ridiculous rate because people aren't going there. But if pubs are going, working men's clubs are going and sports clubs are all integrated, then men don't have that safe space just to be men. This has absolutely nothing to do with equality and integration, but everybody needs a space to just be themselves without having to think about or fear being seen as politically incorrect. Political correctness has become a massive thing, and if you stand against it you don't stand a chance. Being misconstrued as politically incorrect by putting up one's hand and saying, "A female is bullying me. I'm being bullied in the workplace." We know there are male bosses that bully male staff, but female bosses bullying male staff, we never hear of this.

I've had great relationships with other female direct reports, and they've been some of my closest friends, and I've always had great relationships with my male bosses. So I don't know, but it's interesting to read that post-pandemic statistics say that men aren't socialising. And when we take a nasty hard look at our own lives and turn the lens back on ourselves, we realise that most of our male friends are actually the friends of our partners or the partners of our partners' friends. You might look at a party list and say, "Jack's my friend. Well, actually, Jack is Jane's husband. And Jane knows Elizabeth (your partner). So yes, I know Jack. But he's a close acquaintance more than a friend." I think there's a lot to be said for defining things correctly.

The concept of lads' holidays has always been frowned upon, but being able to be silly, or not even silly, but just being in a space where people – men in particular in this instance – can relate is particularly important.

It is always best to stick with it if we can, making sure we've got that support network, that balance, turning it into a piece of armour mentally. Knowing that I lived through that experience, I know I can I do anything that is hard, difficult or that I'm struggling with. Is my mental health as bad as it was? No, I dealt with that. I don't experience any stigma because I don't tell anyone, but when I do have the topic opened, I try and turn it into a positive.

I also don't talk about it because of the stigma, and a really good message to this point is that the reason this is anonymous is because an employer asked me not to go on record because they are afraid of how it would affect their business. It's not fashionable to say such things.

Obtaining a balance is key and can be found in male-only spaces, whether a rugby club or a working men's club – not that there are many of those left, nor the golf clubs, because all of that is being eroded. Perhaps get some drinking buddies, but whatever it is, the key is to get that balance, because if you're at work 9:00 am to 5:00 pm Monday to Friday and you're constantly being told *you're no good, you can't do it, your work's rubbish*, and if you don't have someone saying, "Yeah, come on!" or "Oh, well done!" or someone even just telling you jokes and laughing, then you don't have that emotional levelling. It doesn't have to actually level up. It probably won't, but if you don't have your depleted confidence and positivity topped up a bit out of hours, as it were, then you'll never be able to cope.

Find those male-only spaces if you can, and just do stuff that makes you happy. It's not easy because it takes other people to make you do it, because the first thing you want to do is just hide. Sleep was a great release, and I would try and sleep a lot if I weren't working; that would be my preference because that was safe, that was warm, that was nice. But actually, being dragged out to do stuff was much, much better.

What I would also recommend for those going through any kind of bullying is to hold it in your memory and make it a piece of your armour for the future; dealing with it is one thing, but using it to your benefit afterwards is the next thing. But first of all, you've got to deal with it.

REFLECTIONS

REFLECTIONS

REFLECTIONS

ELEVEN

ANXIETY: ALEX

I've not got a specific date when I became aware of my feelings and the things I was struggling with, but it was right around the time of the 2008 recession. I was fifteen, so right in the middle of my teenage years, those core years where I was developing as a human and becoming a man.

The recession hit my family hard. I wasn't necessarily aware of things bubbling up before that – at thirteen and fourteen you don't really care about all that stuff. But when you start to turn fifteen and sixteen, that's when you start to pick up on things because you become more emotionally aware of what's going on around you. And this fed into the relationship I have with my mum and dad.

I have an incredibly strong and close connection with both my parents and I'm proud of that. It's something I'll always cherish and continue to nurture. My mum is the kind of person who very much wears her heart on her sleeve; she's very emotionally invested in things, so much so that she now works in mental health herself. My dad, however, is a "typical bloke", a very nice guy, really funny, but doesn't talk about his feelings and private stuff.

The thing that stands out to me the most from that time is the anxiety I started to experience when my dad was made redundant out of the blue. My dad has always been the breadwinner, the person that works the longer hours and earns the most money in the household. Obviously during a global recession, that's not the greatest thing, but it is the way things were for my family.

I remember coming home from school the day after Dad got the news. He was sat on the sofa winding down, and he just didn't seem himself. Suddenly he started blurting out things about how he was feeling, and then without warning he started to cry. I'd never seen my dad cry, and I've never seen him cry since, if I'm honest. For my dad to be showing that much emotion and sharing with us what was going on in his mind really hit me hard. Don't get me wrong; it brought me closer to my dad, and I respect him more for sharing himself in that way, but at the same time it made me feel horrendous, like I needed to do something, I needed to act, I needed to help him; and that was the trigger for me.

I know there are a lot of other people out there that will have significantly worse events, but for me that was really a trigger for my overthinking, severe anxiety, and panic attacks. In no way at all am I blaming my dad for it – he was going through a very raw thing, a really challenging time. But that's just how it made me feel.

From that point on, I started to overanalyse and overthink absolutely everything, which fed into every part of my life. It fed into my relationships with friends, with myself, and into my relationship with how I look. I started gaining weight at quite a rapid rate, and this continued throughout university. It got to a point where I was horrendously miserable, and I didn't really have relationships with my friends – they liked me, and I liked them, but I'd always find excuses and ways to not properly interact with them because I was so concerned about what people thought of my appearance.

Now that doesn't necessarily stem from the way I was feeling after my dad was made redundant, but that overthinking and that anxiety led to the way I was. And the problem was that I never changed. I never understood why I felt like that. I never understood why I seemed to think, 'I'm just going to keep eating and just get bigger and bigger.' I understood there was a connection, but I didn't want to go out and build those relationships because I feared what people thought of me.

I know it sounds like a cliché, but I was eating to feel something, because there were times when I was simply numb. I wasn't anxious, I wasn't angry, I was just empty, and eating was a way to feel enjoyment for a few seconds. It wasn't until people pointed it out that I realised I was getting so large.

My social anxiety did get a little bit better through university, and I guess that's a natural progression as you get a little older, and you're almost forced to build relationships. But right around the time I finished university, my grandmother died, which had a devastating impact on me.

When I was young, my mum and dad both worked full-time jobs, so every half term – in fact, at every possible opportunity – I would be at my maternal grandparents' house. My grandparents lived an hour away from us and so I always stayed for a couple of days or a week at a time, which was much easier for my mum and dad, and I always enjoyed it. My grandparents, particularly my grandmother and I, had a deep connection because we were very similar: we shared a sense of humour, similar tastes in food, pretty much everything.

There was something different about the relationship I had with my grandmother. Not that it was better or worse in any way, it was just different. My grandmother was quite a proper lady; she did things by the book, and she was straight-edged. She was also someone I could always talk to, and she consistently showed affection. Even though she wasn't necessarily, on the face of it, the type of woman who was what today we would call empathetic, behind closed doors she was very much that type of woman. As I got older, my relationship with her never changed, whereas sometimes with family members and others, relationships do change, and they need to change.

In 2016/2017 my grandmother had a stroke, and after she was

discharged from hospital, she deteriorated rapidly, so much so that one day my mum went to visit, and twenty minutes before my mum arrived, my grandmother passed away. I believe she'd had another stroke, and, unfortunately, this time it was just a little bit too much. My mum called me and told me the news, and I remember at that point deciding to essentially bury my emotions. I'm quite open in admitting that's what I did because that's what *I chose* to do.

I remember on that day feeling nothing. I was just numb. Cold. Alone. Even though I had people around me.

My mum is incredibly strong mentally, but she's also quite fragile in certain areas; certain things can overwhelm her. In her job, she must be strong for those people that she's trying to help, but for herself, things can get on top of her. Choosing to bury my emotions wasn't necessarily a choice I made to be strong for my mum so she wouldn't see me upset; at the time I thought it was the best thing for me to do. Every day after that I gradually got more and more numb to the situation.

About two years later, I was at work, which was getting on top of me due to the relatively new role I'd taken on. Things had started to spiral, and my work wasn't as good as I knew I could deliver or was expected to deliver.

I didn't have any relationships, and I was just doing the same thing repeatedly. When people asked me if I was okay, I would do the usual, "Yeah, I'm fine, don't worry about it," as so many people do.

But I wasn't fine. I'd buried things for so long that I didn't really know what was wrong with me, and this was making me even more anxious behind closed doors. The anxiety when you don't know why you're anxious is one of the worst, in my opinion. I think it's something that isn't talked about enough, and because you can't answer that question, you don't have the answer to many questions. That's okay, but people need help to find the answers to those unknown questions. I got to a point where I was starting to have panic attacks in the toilets at work, and these weren't small panic attacks; they were full on, to the point I thought I was having a heart attack.

Eventually I spoke to my mum about some of it. I didn't tell her everything, and she said, "Talk to someone." I didn't take her advice. I put it to the back of my mind and the panic attacks combined with the severe anxiety kept happening, to the point where I thought maybe I should just end it.

Now, my story might be a little bit different to those of other people in the sense that I thought that for a momentary second.

I didn't act on it. I didn't attempt to act on it. It was very much a momentary second of a thought I had. And it was at that point that I knew I needed to kick myself into gear. That sounds very simple when it's written here, but it wasn't. It was hard to find the right person to talk to. I wanted to find someone removed from the situation, and I wanted to find someone from a completely neutral background.

I was becoming constantly anxious. I wasn't sleeping. I was having severe panic attacks. I broke down at work a few times, but I still didn't tell people why I was feeling this way or even what I was feeling, because I thought they'd want to get rid of me. I knew the people I worked alongside of and worked for quite well. I made up the story in my own head that they wouldn't want to hear me talk about my problems. There was some truth to it, potentially, but I don't want to paint them as the villain, because they certainly weren't. I thought if I showed this weakness, they wouldn't want me working there anymore. I had no evidence or indication that this would happen; it was just a story I made myself believe.

I spoke with my mum again about bits and bobs, but I missed out lots of things. She gave me the same advice, that I needed to speak to someone. And again, it sounds so simple but it's so powerful. And this is where my story takes a little bit of a turn. I did go and speak with someone. I removed myself from my workplace for no real reason that other people could see, but I just wanted to get out of there.

I had therapy sessions every single week, sometimes twice a week. He didn't really tell me much, he just let me speak and let me get it all out, giving me a little nudge here and there. Not a shove, not a push, just a gentle little tap.

And the biggest thing I learned was that it's absolutely okay. There is nothing wrong with me, you, us … or rather, there *is* something wrong with us all, but it's okay for that to be so.

I guess people now are going to think I'm cured, I'm fine, I'm done, but it's still a battle. It's still a battle as I still have bad days, to the point where it affects my relationships. I become irritable, I become a horrible person to be around, and I have no reason for it, it's just the way my brain works.

I know that I didn't deal with the death of my grandmother, and I still haven't, not properly. I know there are a lot of tragic events out there, but when you don't deal with something, whether it's the passing of a loved one or something else, it will only get worse. It will take time, but if you don't deal with it, it will become a problem, as it is for me.

I wish I could give you a happier ending to this story. I mean, there is a happy ending: I sought help. I went and spoke to someone and I'm quite open about talking about my mental health now. I know there's a lot of good out there for me personally, but there's still a battle that goes on inside my own head. I'm not OK with it, but I'm dealing with it. I'm getting there. And I've learned it's important to understand what someone might be going through. We're not going to know everything about what someone's going through, but we need to listen and understand. I've learnt that those big moments, where you don't feel great … turn them into a series of little moments, smaller obstacles that you need to get over.

Going through something as hard as losing someone so close to me has taught me lessons; it's showed me that I can be weak, and that's okay. It breaks my heart still that she's not with me, especially now that my life is where it is. She's missed a lot of fantastic things that have happened to me, and that's not easy.

I am depressed, but I am okay.

And I'm glad about that.

I went to a very dark place, and I was in it for a long time, and I'm still in it to a certain degree. Maybe we never fully get out of that place, because it leaves scars, it leaves lasting memories – but it's how we deal with those feelings moving forward that's important, that helps us get to a better place. There are still days where it's horrible, but I can deal with them better now.

I never had a proper, strong relationship with a woman before my fiancée, and it's just so good to have a companion. I know a lot of people out there don't have that, but for me, that's what helps me. We don't have to talk about anything, just having her there and being in her presence, as well as my parents' presence, is enough.

Recognising when I need to take myself out of stressful situations both at work and when dealing with things in my personal life, before letting things get on top of me, has been vital. The first step I've taken is speaking to people about my challenges and making sure I let them know where my head is mentally.

In terms of my eating habits and issues with my weight, my fiancée has certainly helped me rein it in a little bit. I have no doubt it was an eating disorder, which I used to numb the pain. My fiancée came into my life at the exact right time. I won't go as far as to say she saved my life, but she definitely kept me on that trajectory that I wanted to be on. I don't feel I need to talk about it too much because she knows how much she means to me, how much she helps my mental health, and she's become someone I can lean on and speak to about things.

I can't say that I ever experience any stigma around what was happening to me, but maybe I was a little bit naive to it at the time because I was so in my own thoughts that I didn't pay attention to anything around me. I was quite a good actor, in the sense that it never got to the point publicly where people were severely worried about me.

When I was at my old workplace, the stigma was in my own head – but I hadn't manifested that out of nowhere; it came from not only the media, but everywhere: *"You're a man. You need to be strong."* All of this anxiety was in my head purely because of the stigma and narrative that is out there, which had seeped into my subconscious more than I realised.

Nowadays, I prioritise self-care by spending time with the people that are close to me, making sure that I'm nurturing my relationships and my friendships. When I'm out playing golf, walking with friends, having a meal with my mum and dad, or watching a movie with my fiancée – those are the times I feel most at peace. Even if you're not talking about anything specific, just being around the people you love is so powerful.

Looking at things from a more logical point of view, without overanalysing and overthinking things, helps me avoid going into a bit of a frenzy. I am not free of my frenzies, as I'm quite an emotive person, and I can get a bit angry, but I'm certainly better at dealing with it as a result of my self-care.

The advice I'd give to anybody going through similar struggles would be to speak to someone. Doesn't matter who it is. I was very lucky that I spoke to my mum, and she gave me some great advice. I can't stress enough how much it helps speaking to someone on a neutral basis, someone who's completely removed from the situation – a therapist, for example.

Saying the words "just speak to someone" sounds like I'm dumbing it down, but I'm not. Life is so simple, but we insist on making it complicated. I know it's hard. I know it's tough … just thinking about it now, I'm getting emotional, but you need to take that step and you'll see how simple it is. Just talk to someone. And keep speaking to people – don't stop after you've done it once.

Keep speaking, vomit everything out! It's so liberating getting it out. Tell people!

People you trust. People you don't even know! You don't have to tell them everything, but just give it a chance.

There's a lot of talk around male mental health and mental health in general now. We are getting to a point where it's being spoken about, but *action isn't being taken*.

The stats on male suicide keep shocking people, so for men to sit down and share their stories together in this book is amazing. I can't say how much joy it fills me with that this platform has grown so exponentially, so quickly, and we're getting to a point now where we're starting to change things. We must keep on that message of *listen* and *understand*.

Things really can change.

REFLECTIONS

REFLECTIONS

REFLECTIONS

TWELVE

REJECTION: ROGER

I'm a happy-go-lucky guy that enjoys life and takes things day by day. My work is enjoyable, and I work hard. I get on well with most people and find people connect with me easily. I'm grateful to have a lot of friends and my closest friends I've known since childhood.

When my wife and I first got married fifteen years ago, we lived in a flat with our two children. Eventually, we moved into a house which we renovated together. I thought we were happy until things started to feel strange. It would be a Monday morning and my wife would ask me if I was going out at the weekend, even though I'd just been out on the Friday and Saturday. I felt as though she wanted rid of me, and I'd say, "I don't know yet" and then wonder why she'd ask such a thing when we had two little girls. Sometimes I wanted to stay in and just play with them. Although they were twins, the bond was stronger with my eldest as there were complications during the birth. One of them stayed with my wife and the other was in neonatal, so I'd go to visit the one in neonatal.

My wife and I were always in the same room throughout the week, as we lived in a flat. When Friday night arrived, I'd finish work, have dinner, and I'd be in the bedroom with the wife in the girls' room playing. My clothes would be laid out on the bed ready to go out, and I'd think, *Well, if you insist!* My mates would say what a great wife I had, "she gets your clothes out, no arguments, you don't need to look after the girls," and I used to think I was so lucky. "Man, you look good," others would say. "You must be living the good life." "I can't complain," I'd say.

Friday would come again, and even though I didn't feel like going out again that week, my wife would encourage me with words such as "Go on, you'll be fine when you're out." So I'd get ready and go out. Sundays would be written off because I was hungover.

At times, I felt resentment because our girls were into gymnastics and I felt they spent all their time there and only needed me to pick them up, like I was their Uber driver. Pick-up times would be around 9:30 pm, and since I'd been up from 4:00 am, sometimes 5:00 am, picking them three times a week up was tough.

Life continued this way, and my work at the time was hard. I had a job that took me all over the country. Bosses came and went, and there was a particular time where I felt a boss had it in for me. I felt he didn't like me for the colour of my skin, although he'd say certainly not. I knew because I had spoken to him on the phone before we actually met, and then he completely changed when he saw my face, so there was no way I was working for someone like that. I didn't let it really bother me until he indirectly threatened my job. I decided to leave, as I felt I was being undermined and I knew I was better than that. My wife wasn't working so all the living expenses were down to me to pay.

I'd been with the company for nearly eight years when a new director arrived, and I felt then I had to start again. It was obvious he didn't want me there, which wasn't a good feeling. I spent most of my day at work, and it needed to be my happy place. I was a chef and good at what I did, so I was always going to find work, which I did.

Even though I was happy in my work life, always laughing and joking, I started to feel sad when I was at home because it was always so quiet. At work, I was able to keep my own schedule so I'd go where I wanted for days or for the week. I'd have little sleep at home and just get up and go to work, and no one questioned that at the time. I'd get in from work about 10:00 pm, go to bed, and by 3:00 am I'd be up ready to work. I felt as though I wasn't wanted in my own home.

When I was at home, I'd just sit watching TV but not really paying attention to what was on, just thinking to myself, 'Is this what it's all about?' I carried on going out at weekends like clockwork for two to three years.

The wife and girls would be at the gym, and if I was at home by myself with the TV and the cats, I would sit and think, 'Bloody hell, I'm just going to work, paying bills and being a taxi.' When I did pick my family up from the gym, there was nothing to say unless we spoke about gymnastics. It'd got to the point where my wife and I just stopped talking completely. The car was silent.

When my wife and I first met we'd talk about anything and everything. I met her as she was walking across the road in Nottingham city centre with a mate I used to go to school with. I stopped in my tracks and said, "I don't know that girl but I'm going to marry her." I didn't see her again for a year, until she was at my cousin's house when I was there. One night on the off chance, we spoke in the kitchen. We didn't know each other, but something in my head told me to grab her, and she hugged me. I think I embarrassed her. After that day we were inseparable. I'd go to work, she'd go to work, and after work I'd drive to hers. We'd talk in the car for hours, sometimes all through the night. Then we'd go to work in the morning, and this continued for a while. I played football at the time, and she was the only girlfriend that was there. We'd go to the pub after the game and be in the pub till nine at night, every weekend. But that was the early years.

One night my breathing started to change, and I could feel my heart beating as if it wanted to pound out of my chest. At one point I thought I was dying. I called out to my wife that I was having a panic attack. She was upstairs bathing the girls. It seemed as though I was shouting at the top of my voice, and no one could hear me. I didn't know what was happening. I just knew something was not right. I remember feeling really sad inside, especially after telling my wife I thought I was stressed, and she didn't really say much.

Shortly after this panic attack, I started to see programmes coming on the TV all about stress. I was recognising signs that were on these programmes as the same things that were happening to me. I talked to my brothers at the time, and one said you need to just get away from it all, so he took me to see my dad in Jamaica for two weeks of relaxation, where I gathered my thoughts and decided on the next chapter of my life.

After this holiday, when I felt myself getting stressed, the first thing I noticed was that my heart rate and breathing would change. I recognised this and was able to calm myself down, first by using breathing techniques I'd learnt or by singing to myself. The levels of stress would always happen when my wife was upstairs and I was alone.

The holiday gave me clarity, and realising how long I'd felt sad was surprising, because I was going to work to pay bills and hadn't realised this had been going on for a few years. When you are in it, you don't realise how much time passes. I had a young family and I felt as though I had to provide for them all. Eventually the wife and I separated, and even though we're still married and close to one another, we had to part.

I noticed I'd lost weight and looked good on the outside, and it felt great. I hadn't gained weight due to the depth of sadness, I just lost a lot, and loved it. I started buying smaller clothes for my body type and looked as though I was going to the gym.

When you are generally a happy person and then feel so sad and worthless on the inside, you need to get help.

All this sadness and stress was a good few years ago, and I know now that when I get stressed the first thing is to talk about it and not bottle it up. It was a scary time, and I don't ever want to feel that way again. I've also learnt that it's good to talk to people. Lucky for me, I realised my signs and had my brothers to talk to and support me. Many people are not so lucky. Stress and anxiety are not healthy, so if you don't feel like you can confide in anyone, you must speak to a professional.

REFLECTIONS

THIRTEEN

FATHERHOOD: NICK

I'm a thirty-seven-year-old man with an average life. I'm a dad, stepdad, and an average electrician ... well, I was until last year when I started working from home. I'm an amateur motorbike racer and just a run-of-the-mill northern chap.

My upbringing was a normal '90s/'00s one in the north of England, Yorkshire to be exact, God's Country as us locals call it. I had a loving family and never really wanted for much as a child growing up. I didn't have any real trauma or problems either; I wasn't bullied at school, and I couldn't ask for better parents, so I can't say that my problems with mental health are due to any of that.

As a child I spent a lot of time with my grandparents as my parents worked a lot doing shifts. This is where I sparked an amazing bond and friendship with my hero, Grandad Frank. And let me tell you, he was some bloke, was Frank. He was a retired miner and a very old-school Barnsley fella, and he was my world, my everything. When I was growing up I hung on his every word, and between Frank and my dad they taught me to be the man I am today.

When I was about eighteen or nineteen, I suddenly fell ill with what I was to find out later was a massive infection that did some damage to my kidneys. This is where my mental health problems started, but I just didn't know it yet. As a nineteen-year-old lad living in the north of England, my social life and friendship circle revolved around going out into town three or four nights a week, and I absolutely loved it.

Barnsley is a small ex-mining town, and everyone knew everyone, so a night out was always good and trouble-free, mostly. When I fell ill with the *E. coli* infection and realised the damage it had done to my kidneys, I had to watch what I was drinking. But I didn't, and this made me even more ill. I didn't have a drinking problem at all, but I loved the social aspect of going out, and then suddenly I had to change my whole social life and circle – everything I knew – which was really hard. I felt like I had to try to reinvent myself.

This was to have a significant impact as time went on, and I still suffer with my kidneys to this day, but I now manage it better and cope with the issues. At the time, I sort of coped. I just limped along and carried on trying different hobbies to find new friendship circles, but I never felt like I fitted in.

On 18 September 2007, at the grand old age of eighty-six, Grandad Frank passed away, holding my hand in the hospital. This hero of mine who I thought was indestructible, who I'd never even seen sad, let alone ill, was gone. I was devastated, and still to this day, as I write this, I do so with a smile on my face and tears in my eyes. I never dealt with the grief, I just helped my family and stayed strong to hold them together and thought, 'I'll deal with it tomorrow', but tomorrow never came.

Dealing with grief was something I'd never had to do and didn't know how to do, so I shut that door to myself and never dealt with it. This was to turn out to be a huge mistake.

A few years later, the best day of my life happened: on 12 March 2016, my son was born, a healthy twelve-pound little boy, Jackson Frank, his middle name after my hero, my Grandad Frank. If you're a dad, you'll know that you get so excited about this moment and then bang, a nurse hands you this tiny little human and you have no clue what to do, because if I'm not mistaken, the instruction manual never came out with him. You just wing it as a dad and hope you can do your best by your child. So, with no instruction manual and a tiny human that relied on me for *everything*, I embarked on a journey of self-discovery and wonderful new smells and sights.

The first fourteen days of being a dad I can honestly say were amazing; it was magical, but I worried about everything. I know if you're a dad reading this, you have done things such as randomly turn the light on in the night to check if your child is breathing, did he have enough milk, why didn't he cry in the last hour, how come he blinked forty times in a minute and not forty-five like the minute before?

Day fifteen was a Saturday and Jackson was grouchy. He wasn't normally grouchy, but he didn't eat much and didn't want to even be touched. There were no other signs that would tell me what was about to happen. I put Jackson to bed in his little cot beside my side of the bed, as normal, and went to sleep. I woke at 3:00 am and my first thought was, why hasn't he woken up for his night feed? He's always awake about 1:00 am for his routine feed.

At this point I flicked on the light and noticed he wasn't breathing, although his throat was moving up and down. Later I'd find out this was called a tracheal tug and was due to the shallowness of his breathing. We immediately rushed Jackson to hospital, and within fifteen minutes of being in A&E he was taken through to resus, and at this point we knew something was seriously wrong. I stood back to see this helpless little fifteen-day-old boy laid on an adult-sized bed with doctors and nurses rushing round him putting needles, tubes, and breathing equipment on him – and my world came crashing down.

After they stabilised Jackson, they gave him a lumbar puncture and quickly found out he had viral meningitis, and later, septicaemia. For a few days, the doctors didn't hold out much hope my little boy was going to make it, and they tried to prepare us for the worst.

I wasn't ready to give up that fight, even though we couldn't even touch him, let alone hug him, due to the pain it caused him. His temperature and heart rate would rocket intermittently, and he had convulsions. I stayed by his side 24/7, reading him stories and just willing him to come home.

Eventually Jackson made a recovery and came home several weeks later. This was a huge trauma I once again never dealt with. I just stayed strong for Jackson and my family, pushing my own emotions down deeper.

When Jackson was two years old, my relationship with his mum broke down and we went our separate ways. It wasn't a messy split, just one of those things; our relationship had run its course, and it was best that we did that, but the thought of not seeing my little boy every day crushed me, and I really started to struggle with my mind at that point.

The first night Jackson stayed away from home with his mum I broke down uncontrollably, like when you're a child and you cry so hard you can't catch your breath.

I realised at this point that I was in trouble but didn't know just how much trouble. I had gone to a place where any normal rational thinking was lost, and I just didn't see the point in being here anymore.

I wasn't needed or wanted.

I grabbed some paper and a pen, wrote a note, and left it on the bed, and then I proceeded to go up into the loft. I grabbed my camping bag and a few bits, made a noose, and packed a bag. I knew a spot in the woods not far from my house where no-one would be and I could do what I needed to do. I was hell-bent on killing myself (I still have the note to this day as a reminder of how far I've come on my journey).

I'd got in my head that my son was with his mum and he didn't need me and certainly didn't need a dad that was a failure like this. I'd really lost the will to keep going. My head was so far gone and full of trauma that I'd snapped and couldn't take any more.

As I started to go downstairs, my dog Marley the Labrador – who was a grumpy, sleepy, gentle old soul – came up the stairs as I was going down and stopped me in my tracks halfway down the stairs, something he'd never done before and never did again after. Marley wouldn't move, no matter how much I begged him, so I just sat crying on the stairs.

As I did, I happened to look up and saw a photo of Jackson at one day old that was hung up on the stairs. I cried and screamed like I never had before – how could I leave my son?

With hindsight, it was at this point that I really should have spoken to someone or tried to get help, but I didn't because I felt ashamed and embarrassed about what I had done and how I was feeling in my own head.

How could I possibly ask for help or talk to anyone about this? I'd never asked for help from anyone, and the one man I needed wasn't here anymore. I was lost, my mind had snapped, and I had nowhere and no-one to turn to. So I did what I'd always done: I buried it deep.

I was tormented by my own thoughts and brain all the time, every day. At night I had night terrors, which I still have now at age thirty-seven. A bit of time passed, and I met the woman who is now my wife.

As you do when you start dating, I put on a happy-go-lucky front, always the joker, but it didn't take Kat long to realise something wasn't right. She asked me about it but didn't pressure me. I kept saying I was fine, I just had a difficult day at work, or I'm exhausted with my kidneys. Anything I could say to put her off and buy me some time before she noticed again. I was in mental turmoil every day. I'd come home in my van and scream or cry before putting the mask back on and going home smiling like nothing was wrong. Kat and I got married, and let me tell you, that was one amazing day. It put a lot into perspective.

A few weeks later, Kat asked if I was okay, and I finally said no, I'm not. But instead of my wife taking this like it was her fault, she was so supportive, and I can't thank her enough. She encouraged me to seek help and was not only my wife but my best friend. I didn't tell her the whole story, only snippets, but I knew I could do this without feeling ashamed.

When I started counselling, I felt like I'd let myself and my family down as a "man", as a father, husband and stepdad, because society builds men up and puts them on this pedestal of being hard, with no emotions: "men don't cry", "men don't show any sign of weakness."

Well, that's total and utter rubbish. I now understand something that my Uncle Ron said to me when I was about fifteen: *"Be strong enough to be gentle, but gentle enough to be strong."*

Counselling, to start with, was hard. I knew it would be good, but I didn't want to accept that I needed it. But it was the best decision I've ever made, and I urge anyone to please, please try it and be open-minded to it when you do go.

After a few sessions, they got me to start writing a diary of all the things that upset me or made me anxious, and it turned out I had a lot of demons! We slowly worked through the past traumas, and it helped me to finally deal with my grief and confront the trauma of my son's meningitis.

All these things that I'd let build up, I started to accept and learn how to control my own mind better. I am still on a journey to recovery – I still have night terrors, I still check on Jackson every night without fail – but I can deal with all this in a much better way. I still have those bad days, but now I don't let those bad days turn into bad weeks and bad weeks into bad months. I have the tools now to help me go forward with my life, and I believe this has made me be a better father, stepdad, and husband.

Life is hard, and life is stressful, and just when you think you have it figured out, it has a funny way of giving you a reality check. If you're reading this and you feel the way I did, please seek help – but make sure it's the right help.

I finally opened up to a friend, a guy I met through racing (unfortunately he's a southerner, but we can't all be perfect!). I was terrified; I mean, up to this point I'd only spoken about any of this to my counsellor, which was a lady over the phone, and my wife, to whom I'd only told bits.

When I decided to talk to Stew, I thought he was going to call me soft or an idiot (stronger words may have been used). I had this in my head that this was how he'd react, but he didn't, he was just incredibly supportive and didn't try to change the subject or call me anything. It was just a normal conversation, and it was a huge light bulb moment for me knowing that talking about this stuff can actually be a normal conversation.

This whole taboo around men not talking needs to stop and needs to change.

Please, I implore you, reach out, because yes, it's a huge step and won't be easy, but it will be the best decision you will make on your journey to recovery.

Opening up to another man was a big step, and I thought it would be the hardest conversation of the ones I'd had, but it turned out to be the easiest.

Since I've had this conversation, I'm in a much better place. I often talk openly to other men about my experiences and depression, and you'd be surprised how many men reciprocate with their own stories of how they've suffered or are currently suffering, that I had no clue about.

The journey has been the most difficult and darkest one I have ever experienced, but now I have the tools to help me, and I can spot and pick up when I need some intervention, be that from my support network or just myself.

I regularly take time to myself, building Lego or listening to an audiobook. This helps give my mind the time and space to relax and puts me in a better frame of mind to process a trigger or experience that previously would have sent me into a depressive episode.

I've started a podcast talking about my experiences and helping other men talk. This has been a huge step, as talking about it openly was hard, but the feeling I had afterwards was near on euphoric. It's a hard feeling to explain. Yes, I was exhausted, but it was a massive weight shift for me personally.

If I have one piece of advice for anyone who is suffering from mental health issues or is having a difficult time, it would be to talk; just pick up the phone or ask a friend or relative to talk.

Don't give up if the first person you talk to isn't in the right space or doesn't have the right mental attitude themselves and can't help. Seek out the right advice and the right help – like the people at Tough to Talk, who are doing an amazing job helping men.

Together we can break this stigma, and men can stop suffering in silence.

REFLECTIONS

REFLECTIONS

FOURTEEN

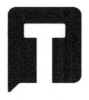

INCEST: RYAN

My life has never been okay.

My childhood wasn't the greatest, growing up with the person I'm going to call "father" – and know that's the only time I'll ever use the word "father".

He wasn't the best, and he wasn't around a lot anyway. But when he was, he was controlling, narcissistic, and beat the hell out of Mum if he didn't get his own way. Growing up, we knew from an early age we had to do whatever he wanted just to keep the peace.

As far as I was concerned, I thought that was what every family structure was, because when other people were around and he was there, he was a completely different person. There were niceties, but as soon as the front door shut behind guests, that's when the dynamics changed. I just assumed in other people's houses it was the same.

It wasn't until later in life that I realised that wasn't the case.

Growing up, me and my brother didn't have the best of times. I had a bit more of a social life as a child, always outside playing football and other games with friends, but my brother Kevin was such an indoors kind of child that he witnessed more abuse than I did. And he experienced more.

He had a much worse time than me.

He'd see a lot more and would feel the wrath of the person we referred to as "SD", for "sperm donor", and will forevermore.

We stayed with him until I was about eleven and Kev had just turned fifteen. I honestly believed every family dynamic was like ours, so when my mum said that we were leaving him, I wondered why. I didn't understand. All my friends lived nearby, and I really didn't want to go, but obviously I went.

We moved around a couple of times after leaving SD, and then settled down somewhere. When we'd visit SD, I noticed his true behaviour even more, finally seeing the way he'd treated my mum, trying to control her and make out that she was worthless.

It wasn't the best of times, and when I was about eleven or twelve, my mental health problems started to show at school. That's when I started going to counselling at school and had no idea why I needed it. I was in there with lots of different counsellors, because the problem back then, and I guess it's still the same now, is that if you go to a regular counsellor, which you get referred to by the doctor, they only give you so many sessions. I always found that once I'd reached the end of each session, I felt better about myself. You go back, but you're not really fixed. Then you go back into counselling again and have to start back at the beginning.

Nowadays, I wonder why they can't continue using your notes, see where you got up to, so they can give you a more positive end experience, getting to the crux of things.

School life wasn't great because SD was always in the papers for being a peeping Tom, stealing money from the local council and things like that; and because we lived on an island which was only thirty-two miles round, everyone knew our business. His stuff was in the local paper, which the kids at school read, which made school life hard. When I was about to take my GCSEs, *The Star* national newspaper picked up on a story of him working as Father Christmas in a Christmas grotto.

For some reason, he'd come back to the island and went down the local paper printing place where you can give them your stories. He was doing this because he thought he was untouchable. He could do whatever he wanted. Everyone loved him.

And because the local press had loads of knowledge on him, they knew he was doing wrong. They contacted the national press, and that's when it appeared in *The Star*, just when I was doing my GCSEs.

It was hard seeing it in the press, a big picture of him dressed up as Father Christmas, and all the kids would look at me and laugh. I don't know if it was just my mind thinking that they laughed at me or if I was just assuming they were laughing at me; they could have been laughing at something completely different.

I still went to see him at the weekends up until I was nineteen, mainly so I could try and stop mum getting abuse from him, and so I could see my friends who I grew up with. I never understood why Kev never went to visit him, but I found out later in life.

Staying at his flat one evening, he put himself upon me and did stuff to me that no father should ever do to their son; and when I tell people that, the number of questions I've had to answer … including, "Well, you were nineteen, you should've known better. You should know it's wrong. You know you should've fought him off", and yes, I should have, but growing up we'd been conditioned to always do what he wanted just to keep the peace. And to be honest, I just froze and let him do what he wanted so I didn't get beaten up, get more grief and my mum didn't get any more abuse. I was protecting myself and my mum.

I remember leaving his flat and driving home just crying all the way home. But I knew that I couldn't say anything to anyone because I thought, "Who will believe me? Who? Who's gonna believe that a father would do anything like that to their son?" So I kept quiet for about seven years.

Then as I was turning twenty-six, I was due to get married, and I thought to myself, 'We're going to spend the rest of my life together, so I'm gonna be open and honest for the first time about it.' So I told her, and she gave me the confidence to tell my mum.

It broke her heart. And then she said, "Well, you've got to ring Kev."

He was living in London at the time, so I rang him, and that's when we found out that between the ages of five and fifteen, it had been happening to him repeatedly.

His words to me were, "I went through all of that so it didn't happen to you." That just broke me. I felt like I'd let him down. I felt like he'd gone through all that for nothing. We had a long chat on the phone and his decision was that he didn't want to do anything about it. He'd moved on, dealt with it in his own way. We didn't know the way that he dealt with at the time, but later in life he told us he had drunk lots, done drugs and prostituted himself to random men, because as far as he was concerned, that's what love was. So we didn't do anything about it.

When I got married and had my first child, I tried to have a normal life, and then I found out Kev had been diagnosed with hepatitis and full-blown AIDS due to all the sleeping around and the things that he'd done. At this point we knew he wouldn't have a long life, as this is going back to 2005 was when my eldest was born, and medicine since then has completely changed.

Kev told us he was going away to Manchester for a week to meet some friends, and I went to work on the Saturday morning, and I got a call from my wife at the time telling me we'd a weird voicemail from Kev saying, "Ryan, help me, help me. I don't know where I am. I need you. Help." I told her to ring back and see what was going on, so she did, and then rang me telling me it was Manchester police. They told her that he'd told them he'd been date raped by three men and ended up walking the streets at 3:00 am, battered and bruised. The milkman had picked him up and taken him to the police station.

We drove all the way to Manchester to get him, and he came to stay with us. He was really ill, vomiting everywhere.

This was the point at which things between me and Kev changed.

He'd always been the big brother, and now I was the big brother. I was looking after him. During the investigation, the Manchester police found out what had happened in the past, and they said that they needed to take it further. This is when I contacted our local police on the island, and we took Kev all the way back to where we used to live, with the police coming to speak with us both separately and unofficially. We both gave a statement, but we had to do a formal statement a couple of weeks later, as we were now in a place to take action against SD.

I'd already given my statement and Kev was due to come back to do his, but, unfortunately, he got admitted into hospital because he now had gastric enteritis. I called to speak with him on the Thursday, then rang him on the Sunday morning at ten o'clock as I was going to work. I said, "How you feeling?" He said, "I should be home today or tomorrow." I replied, "Great, brilliant. Well, you know, when you're feeling better, we can get you back down here and you can do your official statement." He agreed to this and we finished the call.

At 10:15 am the doctors and nurses found him dead on the floor of the hospital. They said he'd died instantly from a brain aneurysm. They managed to start his heart again. I don't know how they got hold of Adam, his boyfriend, but he drove from London to the island to pick up me and my mum, back to the London hospital where Kev was. None of us knew why, but the hospital rang a couple of times and said, "Are you on your way?" I responded, "Yeah, we're just stuck in traffic because, as you know, it's not an easy journey."

I knew something wasn't right, so when Mum asked me who was on the phone, I just said, "It's Kev asking the hospital to ring us." I knew I couldn't say the truth. We got to the hospital and saw Kev with all these tubes attached to him. We asked, "What's happened?" We asked if we could go over and see him, to which the doctor replied, "No, but please follow me into my office."

Sitting there, we were told what happened: "His brain swelled so much that it couldn't go any further, so the swelling started working its way down the spinal column." I'd never heard of that before. If he survived, he'd be a vegetable, just a body lying there without being able to do anything.

That's something you never want to hear, so we sat around his bedside all night whilst the doctors were doing tests. We called some of his friends from London to come and be with him, and it was the most beautiful but strange evening, with us all sitting there laughing and just sharing stories of Kev. He was lying there, this shell of who he used to be, with the machine making his body pump blood around his body. The doctors continued to do tests; they would come in and lift his eyelids, and you could see there was no life there. You'd see the eyes looking at you, but there was nothing there.

I tried to give mum hope, that there was a chance, but I knew there wasn't. I think she realised it, but she didn't want to admit to it. In the morning, the doctors pulled us into this other room, and said, "We're sorry, but there's nothing else we can do. Do we have your permission to switch the machine off?"

That was the hardest decision for mum to ever have to make, to give that permission to end her son's life, even though technically he'd already gone. We agreed, and said our final goodbyes before they turned the machines off. Everything just drained from him. We stayed for a while, said our goodbyes and then we left the hospital.

We called the police to say that Kev had passed away. We'd been told that just on Kev's statement alone, if he'd made the formal one, SD would be looking at fifteen years' jail time minimum, and that was without my statement.

By this time, the law had changed so that they could use cases from other times someone had been to court for different things. We found out that the worst sentence he'd ever got, which we didn't know about, was a two-year suspended sentence. With this case, our case and other cases, there was a massive case against him.

I asked the police, "Well, what happens now? Because obviously Kev's statement's not valid." They said, "Look, we can still go ahead on yours, and use Kev's as an unofficial one as a character witness."

I'd just lost Kev so there was no way I was gonna stop this now. I wanted justice for Kev's life. So I went to the magistrates' court, walked in and was escorted out because I wasn't allowed to be there. The case got sent to the Crown Court, as it was now turning into a huge case. A couple of days before the case was supposed to happen, I was invited to the court to familiarise myself, because I was anxious about it – not because of the retelling of what had happened but because of being questioned by the defendant's team and them making us all out to be liars.

The day after the tour of the court, I got a call from our local hospital asking if I was Ryan, and I replied, "Yeah, what is it?" And they replied, "We believe we've got your father here."

"What do you mean?"

"Well, he's been admitted as he's got a brain tumour. He's only got twenty-four hours to live."

I didn't believe it at first. I thought to myself, "This is him trying to get out of it somehow." Then, I don't know why, but I asked, "Can I come and visit him?" to which they agreed.

My wife at the time drove me to the hospital. The head nurse pulled us into her office, and I explained the situation and I told her, "I want to see if it's him."

She responded, "You can do it, but he's unconscious. He can hear you, but he can't talk." This to me was perfect.

Walking up to his cubicle, I stood at the end of his bed and just looked at him. I pulled the curtains around us because he was in the ward with other people, and I thought, 'This is my time.' Sitting down beside him, I said everything I wanted to say. Everything that he needed to hear about what I was going to say in court.

Then I just got up and left.

I didn't say goodbye.

Or "I forgive you" or anything.

In the early hours of the next morning, I got a call from the hospital saying he'd passed.

I cried, not tears of him being gone, of sorrow or emotions of

"Oh, no, I've just lost my dad." But tears of regret and frustration because I thought, 'He's got away with it.'

That's when my spiralling out of control started.

My wife and I had our second child just under a year after Kev passed, and I'd gotten to a point where I couldn't deal with life.

I started being a complete asshole. I had an affair, which ruined the marriage. I lost my kids, started sleeping around, drinking, taking drugs, everything. This went on for about six years. I just didn't care about anyone anymore.

In 2017, my mum managed to get me into a mental health clinic, and they diagnosed me with borderline personality disorder, which I'd never heard of before. They explained that it's to do with the fact that you can't control your emotions, that everything's heightened, and it's brought on by trauma.

I explained everything that had gone on in the past, and she said it might have been there anyway, but the trauma I'd experienced had made it one hundred times worse than what it could've been.

She offered me group therapy courses, and this was the biggest turning point that I needed in my life. The therapy courses gave me the opportunity to look at myself and where I went wrong and deal with stuff that had happened in the past.

Whilst I was doing them, I started training for the London Marathon and ran it in 2017, 2018 and 2019. I started writing my book which was published in 2019.

Ever since then, I've been working and getting my book out there, doing talks to share my story, to help others. I tell them that it doesn't matter what you go through, you know there's always a chance that you can turn it around.

If you believe in yourself and get the right opportunities, get the right help and get people to listen to you, that makes a huge difference.

Getting someone to listen to you and not judge you for who you are, or what you've been through or are going through, is vital.

I lost loads of friends during my downward spiral because I just pushed everyone away. I was this miserable, angry person all the time. I didn't care about anyone else apart from myself, and that was the first time I'd ever really done that. I've always been a people pleaser.

Going from a people pleaser to the most selfish prick you could ever think of is going to push those away who benefitted from your people pleasing.

I never thought I'd be like that, but I just didn't care about anyone else's feelings. Unless I was making myself happy, I didn't care. The truth is I wasn't happy. I thought I was, but I was always looking for that affirmation, for validation, because I thought I had to be in relationship or be with someone to be happy.

I was so wrong, and lockdown was a time that made me happy because I had to be on my own, and I looked into myself even more. I reflected on the group therapy I'd had, and there were still bits there that I hadn't kind of put the pieces together. Lockdown forced me into that situation where I couldn't be around people; I had to be on my own.

I had to build relationships back up with friends and family. It hasn't been easy, but the way I look at it now is that the people I've lost don't deserve me as I am now. I believe that people come into your life for a reason. The right ones stay for a long time. The wrong ones stay for a good time. I've learned that the hard way.

During my struggles with mental health, especially during the recovery and understanding of what's going on, I've experienced stigma and discrimination, especially being a male with mental health issues and me being so open and honest about it.

I felt I got treated completely differently to other people. In one of my jobs, which I was in for twenty-two years, I worked alongside an alcoholic. The bosses bent over backwards for him, especially on a Monday when he'd call up and say he wasn't feeling well. We knew he'd had a drinking session over the weekend, and yet they swept it under the carpet. When I had a meltdown at work once, I started punching a few boxes. No harm to anyone else, but someone saw me do it and went upstairs. The bosses called me up to their office and they said, "If you're caught having another meltdown at work, we'll send you home full pay, and there'll be an investigation."

I responded with, "You know everything that's gone on, you know that I can't help these things, and now you're putting more pressure on me to control something that I can't control just so I can keep a job. You'll bend over backwards just to excuse the alcoholic and not give him any discipline for it, but you're warning me over something that I never chose to have in my life. I never chose to go for that trauma. I never chose to have this illness. You treat me completely differently to someone who chooses to drink to cope with his problems."

I also had to work extra hours to cover the time I went to the group therapy sessions, and yet when people go to the dentist, they'll let them off for that hour. My question is: How is that different?

I'd worked for them since I was nineteen, around the same time SD did what he did to me, and I left in 2019. They witnessed a lot of stuff – when I lost my brother, when I had my affair – and I never kept anything from them.

I never had their support, and I felt like I was a joke to them. They wanted me out of there, but they couldn't sack me because I'd have sued them for unfair dismissal. They were trying to force my hand to get out of there, which I did in the end, so I took redundancy. That's what helped me finish the payment so I could do my book.

Their biggest challenge, and it was their challenge, was that I was a man who was being open and honest about all these feelings about what had happened. I felt like I was treated differently, and I didn't like it.

Sadly, that's not uncommon.

I now prioritise my self-care to help my mental health journey by giving myself space and time if I'm feeling like I don't want to do something, or I'm feeling down. Now instead of forcing myself to do something, I give myself that break. I say, "I'm just not going to do anything today." I spend some time with my girlfriend, but I don't get stressed out and think, "Well, I have to be as normal as everyone else."

I still have a normal life and accept that there will be days when I can't function. I've given up thinking about what the world expects from us as men and feeling like I still must prove myself.

These days it's a case of "I've gotta give myself that time." I give myself that permission and space so I can deal with what's going on, and thankfully, I have fewer bad days now. My anxiety and stress don't happen as often, and I can recognise it nine out of ten times before it happens.

Looking back on my journey, the advice I'd give to somebody who may be going through similar struggles with their mental health and, obviously, with the trauma they've suffered, is this:

Mostly just talk and speak up.

Don't bottle everything up.

Don't think you're less worthy as a human being by admitting to someone that something has gone wrong in your life or you're not feeling right.

There are so many people out there who put on a brave face to please the rest of the world while they're fighting the demons, and that's not healthy.

I truly believe listening saves lives.

If you can find someone who's going to listen to you and not judge you on what you've got to say or what you've been through, that's going to make a huge difference.

If you can be the person who is going to listen without judgement, that can save that person's life. They're going to have this weight lifted off them, feel that they managed to get something off their shoulders, feel like they were not judged or that what happened was questioned. The feeling of 'Wow. Now I'm in a space that perhaps I can deal with that a bit easier. Now I can go and get the help' – that's vitally important.

I know there's help out there, but it's so hard to get these days because it's underfunded and it's still not talked about as much as it should be. There's still a long way to go when it comes to mental health, especially in men.

I believe that men need more understanding when it comes to mental health. We must let go of the expectations of men to be this stiff-upper-lip, tough man who has no feelings.

We say, "Just be who you are." And that must go for everyone. I'll admit it, and I'm not ashamed to say, I'm a mummy's boy, and I've always been that kind of feminine, softer kind of guy. I am not a fighting guy who gets aggressive; even when I did all the drink and drugs, it still wasn't me to be a fighter. I'm more of the "lover, not a fighter" type of guy. And I'm okay with that.

There need to be more men who speak up and say, "I am not a manly man; I can talk about how I feel. I can have bad days, I'm *allowed* to have bad days, I'm allowed to cry."

I think crying makes a huge difference. If you can have a good cry, that's great. I don't cry now because I've cried it out. But years ago, I used to cry all the time and it made a huge difference. It gave me that much-needed release in a way that's necessary.

My experiences with mental health struggles shaped my personal growth and proved to me how resilient I am and how much I wanted to give up in the past, but never did.

I used all that negativity and turned it into power to try and change the world. To make a difference, to put myself out there and say, "This is me, this is what I've been through", because I know there are going to be some people out there who will think, 'If he can do it, I can do it. I can go and talk about it. I can do this; I can do that.'

I think I've turned everything around, and it's weird to admit it, but I'm kind of glad I went through all that stuff because it's made me who I am.

This is the reason why I feel I'm here on this earth. To do this, to share my story, to help just one person. And then it's made it all worthwhile.

I'm continuing to prioritise and manage my mental health in the long term and moving forward to carry on doing what I'm doing. Realising when I'm having a bad day, I can take a step back and look at things, train in the gym so I have positivity going forward, and I have my book out there now. I'm also talking to someone about making a documentary, so I'm trying to raise funds to make it happen.

I was such a quiet kid, and now you can't shut me up. I love talking about my story, even though it's a sad story, but for me I love it because I can go to people who didn't give me the time of day and to the people who thought I'd never amount to anything, and I've achieved more than others could ever dream of.

I'm not saying that in a big-headed or arrogant way, but I feel like I'm a better person than they can ever be because I know 90 per cent of people couldn't go through all that and turn out like this. I think all of them would give up or they'd just go down the wrong path and into crime.

It is important for people to know there's a different way, and there's a reason why people are the way they are, and we mustn't write them off or dismiss them.

When we're having a bad day, we must remember we have to show up, be there, and yes, we're having a bad day, but we're okay we get through the day.

Anything to do with mental health, start talking, because once you start and you know how much better you feel, you can keep going.

Nowadays, I just start talking about my story and I know I'm feeling better because I'm talking about everything. I know everything I'm passionate about, and it brings me back to where I want to be. If I'm going out to a normal day at work, that's a lot harder because that's mundane and boring on a good day. When I'm in a dark place I don't switch off completely, but I tone myself down a bit, just so I can do what I need to do to get through that day.

If I get too bad, then I just don't go in to work that day. I'll just ring up and say, "Look, I'm having a mental health day." I'll be open and honest with them and anyone I come across.

Other than talking to someone, it's so important to be honest. These days I don't see the point in pretending to be someone that I'm not, because that always comes back and bites us. I did that for years, pretending to be something that I wasn't, and it didn't get me anywhere. It got me fake friends, and then when I went for the group therapy and found out who I really was, they didn't want to know me anymore because I was becoming the real Ryan, not this fake one I'd been pretending to be, and they couldn't handle that.

So find the right people and talk, get therapy, train for a sporting event like the London Marathon, or write a book. Be the real you so the right people for you can find you.

REFLECTIONS

REFLECTIONS

FIFTEEN

PSYCHOSIS: SAM

I'm thirty-seven years old and live in Guernsey in the Channel Islands. I have a pretty complex mental health journey that I'd like to share with you.

Life has been a storm from an early age. When I was ten, my auntie passed away with cancer. Shocked, saddened and trying to deal with this, just one year later my dad passed away with leukaemia. He experienced some extremely uncomfortable circumstances prior to his death, and these traumatic memories will live with me forever. Life was tough but I was brushing things aside living as a young child. My uncle – my dad's brother – had lost his wife and his brother, and I believe he didn't know where to turn. As many of us do at tough times, we turn to drugs or alcohol to numb problems and losses in life, and he became addicted to alcohol. I watched as his life unravelled for many years – losing houses, getting into debt, drinking (in my opinion) to numb the pain. After many years, and having his legs amputated as a result of the alcoholism, he passed away from a heart attack. My grandparents had now lost both their sons, whilst still having a number of years left in their own lives. It was incredibly tough to watch.

I left school and became self-employed at the age of seventeen. We set up a garden maintenance business in 2003, my stepdad and me. Mum had remarried by this time to a wonderful man and stepfather that I'm incredibly fortunate to have. He guided me in business and in life, so I had a father figure to inspire me. I worked hard to distract myself from the realities of life's storm and keep going mentally sound and strong.

My other passion in life was football. Football provided me with the exercise and release of endorphins I needed to survive anything thrown my way. As I get older, I genuinely believe that what we need to survive our mental health journeys is someone with relatable life experience who can share *hope* with us and reassure us things will be okay, that we are not alone in our circumstances. Someone else has walked in your shoes and come out the other side. Finding this and understanding this at such a young age was almost impossible. I had no choice; work, family and friends, football ... just keep going!!!

I was married at the age of twenty-two and went on to have two amazing boys who are now thirteen and nine years old. I had everything a young man could dream of: a successful business, my own home, supportive friends and family, an incredible wife, and sons. Life was all going in the right direction, and I had earned the right to captain the Guernsey Football Club as we entered the UK non-league football pyramid in 2011. Seven years passed, and I was living the dream, the closest I would get to being a professional footballer. But during this period, our club physio developed motor neurone disease. All my life I had reached out for father figures, having lost my father and my uncle, and our physio was one of those father figures. Watching him pass away within a two-year period of being diagnosed was heartbreaking and brought back some the traumas of losing my father. My gran had developed dementia through these years and, sadly, passed away, along with my grandfather, who had heart failure after a couple of heart operations. So I experienced the loss of yet more family to different illnesses, and these experiences would stick with me forever.

In 2017, work was good, football was great, but the shit storm of life was about to hit new levels, having already battered me for many years. My wife made it very clear she was no longer happy in our marriage and decided that we should separate. FUCK!!! The stability I had from my family unit, all I'd wanted from a young age, was about to be ripped from under my feet. I agreed things were not great; I admitted that, but we men tend to brush things under the carpet and just hope things will get better. I moved out, living out of a suitcase in my childhood bedroom at my parents' house away from the family. "What the fuck has my life become?" I remember asking myself on many occasions. The breakup of the family at the time was devastating, not least because I had fantastic in-laws, who I'm still close to even now.

In 2017 I also decided to hang up my football boots for Guernsey and call it a day. I couldn't see myself playing any longer with the split custody of my children and my family unit broken, and, to be honest, my body was starting to struggle. Although my wife was one hundred per cent supportive of me continuing to play, and that we would make it work, I felt it was selfish of me to continue allowing football to dictate our lives as it had done for many years. I met with the manager, and his words were, "Be careful. After the highs of many years of football, you could find yourself low and depressed with all that's going on." As it turned out, he was completely right.

I realise now just how much I was struggling – I wasn't talking to anyone about my problems, and I was getting stuck in my own head. One day I found myself strimming some garden banks and crying my eyes out uncontrollably. I called my mum and said, "I can't do this anymore, I need to go to the doctors." I opened up to the GP, and she explained I was experiencing depression – the shock of the marriage breakup and the tragic losses of so many people in my life had caught up with me in my head. And suddenly stopping the hard, physical exercise that football had provided me for many years had impacted my mental health massively.

I was prescribed an antidepressant to get my journey in life back on track. It was a start, anything to help. I hadn't taken a tablet for years, not even a paracetamol. Reluctantly I started the process, and it did give me a serotonin boost, but only after about six–eight weeks of taking it. Straight from the doctors I reached out to one of my football coaches, another father figure who had coached me from the age of seventeen. He's a life coach, works in the fitness industry and has an MBE for the charity work he's done over the years. An absolute legend. I'm thirty-three at this point, and he knows me and my family inside out. "I'm fucked, life is beating me," I told him as I explained the situation I was stuck in. He listened, he supported, and he said openly, "I don't have the answers, Cockers (my nickname), but I can give you some guidance and some tools that can support you."

At this point I hadn't exercised for a couple of months. I left our coffee meeting and headed home to my parents' house. He'd inspired me … and so I ran. I ran to the end of the fairy ring in Guernsey, in the driving rain, got to the end of the cliffs, did press-ups until I couldn't lift myself off the ground, then at the top of my voice I told the world to "FUCK OFF!!" I ran back to my car, then home, and started planning work for the week. With the focus now on fitness, we trained one-on-one. The boxing pads were out, weights, rowing machine, treadmill, and we smashed it to test me to the extreme and release those endorphins. I weaned myself off the antidepressants with the guidance of the doctor and managed to go medication-free for a period. Exercise along with the medication, it all helped and put me in a better place … but I wasn't out of this shit storm yet.

I found myself reaching out to people in different ways to try find people that could relate to my life troubles. Then I discovered Man Club, which I'm still involved with now. It's a space where men talk – or just listen – confidentially and without judgement. We aim to prevent suicide in men and support those going through a difficult time in life through sharing our life experiences. I wish my uncle had had something like Man Club when he was struggling. I believe it could have saved his life. It was in its early stages when I joined, with three or four guys meeting, talking and listening in one of the guys' living rooms. The first time I went, shitting my pants, I arrived at the door of the building and thought, 'Fuck, I'm here.' Not only did I attend, but after listening to a couple of the others speak, I decided, "Fuck this shit! I'm gonna open up and talk!"

At Man Club Guernsey we use a talking stick, which gives the individual who's holding it the power to speak to the room without interruption. I was in control. Well, the whole lot came out, all the tears were shed, a round of applause was given and I gave the talking stick back. Oh my god, did I feel a weight off my shoulders! The feedback from the group was immense; I had made friends for life in an instant! Little did I know this mental health journey wasn't over yet and was ready to throw a massive curve ball at me.

Man Club began a sea swimming group, Numb Nuts, Thursdays at 7:00 am, all year round. The winters were brutal, but sea swimming became our regular meet along with Man Club sessions. The after-effects of sea swimming are incredible; try it if you can. It's now part of my very full mental health toolbox. Brutal exercise was continuing with my life coach and sea swims, and I'd started playing a bit of football for a local club. Things were not in too bad a place.

As I said, I'd moved back into my parents' in my old childhood bedroom, but when they moved to a new, much smaller, house that needed renovating, it was really unsettling for me. I left for work on a Tuesday morning with no idea where I was going at 4:00 pm when work finished. I hadn't seen the house, being wrapped up in my own bubble of confusion trying to get by one day at a time.

I was seeing my boys regularly, so things were good there, but my head wasn't always with them with so much going on. I trained hard, was physically strong, and at this point our family home had been sold and I had found the perfect new house for me and my boys. Over the years my wife and I had renovated our house, converting a garage, and this had added value to our property. We came out of a sad situation selling the family home with equity for each of us. Every cloud has a silver lining and all that. I cheekily spoke to the developers of the new house, whom I knew, and we did a deal on the price of the new house in the unfinished kitchen, and they handed me the keys before a penny had been paid or a paper had been signed. "Cockers, we want to help you out, you deserve this break." My profile in sport meant that my mental health journey in life was well known at this point.

For another ten months I watched my house being built one step at a time, and in November 2018 I bought my new home. The stress relief was insane; I'd worked *so* hard to succeed ... and life settled nicely for a while.

Until one weekend when I went off to Herm, a little island just off Guernsey, to party. I've never smoked or taken an illegal drug in my life – Carlsberg and antidepressants are my only drugs. But this weekend produced what I can only describe as a euphoric experience, which built over the coming days, becoming uncontrollable at times. I was able to find reality in split seconds, gaining some control, but one minute I'd be crying my eyes out, the next I'd be feeling invincible, like I could fly or swim the English Channel!

On the Monday I didn't go to work. I woke up and decided, "I'm not working in my trade today." Looking back, I believe this was the day I fell out of love with garden maintenance. I was high as a kite; I had all sorts of number sequences and patterns recorded in my phone connected to coloured heart emojis; I was convinced I was invincible and could see suicide in people around me. I know now, looking back on it, that it was actually me that was at risk of taking my own life because I felt so invincible.

I picked my boys up on the Tuesday, erratic as fuck. By this point I was hitting what I now know was psychotic mania! But at the time, it all seemed so real – I was hearing voices, I was unsteady on my feet as I tried to look after my children, I was getting flutters in my right ear and a shiver all up my right side. I raced up to my parents' house, where I immediately tried explaining my number patterns and coloured heart emoji sequences ... my parents were blown away, confused as hell about what was going on. I left their house and headed to mine with the kids, and then the mania kicked in big time –

I froze, I couldn't enter my house and the voices in my head were extreme.

I threw the kids back in the car and headed back to my parents'. Distracted by the colour red, I followed the taillights of a car to a property, pulled into the drive, and when the owner stepped out the car asking "Can I help you?", reality hit me for a brief second. "I'm terribly sorry, I'm at the wrong house." I drove out and we headed off to watch the sunset. In the patterns I'd created in my suicide prevention strategy, the orange-coloured heart emoji represented the sunset: "Watch the sunset! It brings joy!" When we got to the headland at Lihou Island, I was hypermanic with psychotic symptoms. There was someone flying a fucking drone, the buzzing was relentless and all my senses were heightened.

Then one of my boys said, "Dad, do you think you could swim to Lihue Island?" "Yeah, no problem, boys!" I was seriously considering doing it, even though I know there's a rip current that would sweep me out to my death. Reality checked in and I raced back to my parents' house with the boys, banging maniacally on the doors and windows to get in. They called my life coach who I'd been training with, and when he arrived I tried to explain what was going on in my head, but it just wouldn't flow. He wanted to get me to the doctors, but I was determined I was going back to Herm the next day ... I promised to go to the doctor when I got back.

That night I slept at my parents'. My children were picked up by their mum and taken safely home with her. At this point, due to the mania, I was sleeping about three hours and had been for a number of days. One important factor with my mental health is sleep – I need plenty and I was having very little! Up at the crack of dawn, everyone concerned for my well-being, I headed off to the bathing pools for a sea swim and to watch the sunrise. The blue-coloured heart emoji represented sea swimming in my depression prevention theory, the yellow heart emoji represented sunrise ... you get my drift. Manic, driving there it felt like every obstacle was in my way, roads shut, lights red, but I made it to the boat after my swim, then off to Herm I went.

The voices in my head were coming back, and when I arrived on the boat I was met by a whole school year group going on a camping trip – the worst scenario imaginable when you have voices in your head. "Can you jump off the boat?" I heard at one point. I considered doing this. Without really realising it at the time, I was the most vulnerable I'd ever been in my life, and I was alone on a boat on my way to an island away from home.

We set sail and I got chatting to another passenger on the boat, a guy in a blue T-shirt. I don't remember his name, but in my eyes he was suicidal and depressed, so I talked to him for the whole journey. We docked and he tried to leave. We shook hands, but I wouldn't let go. I was scared to be alone at that point. Getting off the boat, I decided to help unload the luggage. Fuck knows why, but I did, hauling bags up the gangway with the team from Herm Island thinking, 'Who's this nutter helping us shift baggage!?' The final bag went up, and the guy at the bottom of the run looked distressed. "Are you okay?" I asked. "You go up the steps, I'll come up last." My fear was that he was suicidal, ready to jump in the sea!

I ran around Herm like a man possessed, bumping into various people along the way, till I was stopped and questioned about what I was doing there, and I wasn't insured to be helping shift luggage, etc. This was when a breakthrough came, and Herm Island staff and my football coaches saved my life before I did something tragic.

The week before, I had worked at my other football coach's tent pitch. I explained, "I'm insured to be here, as I worked here last week using your digger and had filled out paperwork." Soon enough, they made contact with my football coach, explaining they had me on Herm behaving erratically, and they were concerned for my well-being. I was guided back to the boat, went back to Guernsey and was greeted by both my football coaches – one being my life coach – explaining I must now get some help because I was not well. To receive psychological help in Guernsey we have to go to Accident and Emergency first to be assessed. In I went, high as a kite, mania controlling my brain and convincing me at times that there was nothing wrong with me. A psychiatrist assessed me, and the conversation must have gone along the lines of "Get him sectioned and up to the mental health ward immediately." I was happy as a pig in shit, laughing and joking like nothing was wrong. We walked round the corner up to the Oberlands Centre, in through the doors and BANG!!! The doors shut, and at this point I was sectioned for twenty-eight days, suffering from psychotic mania caused by bipolar disorder, which I was later diagnosed with.

I refused medication for two days whilst in hospital, determined to fix myself, causing distress on the ward, smashing down the kitchen doors with two water butts, the police pinning me down twice while I was injected with drugs to calm me down! However, at no point did I direct my frustrations or anger at any of the staff. They were amazing with me.

I refused medication because of a heart condition I had at the age of twenty-two. I had severe heart palpitations when I was exercising and needed an operation. The Guernsey doctors prescribed me some medication at the time, and the specialists in London questioned why I was on this medication. I didn't trust the professionals to give me the right tablets again! Finally, I accepted meds, one that was a mood stabiliser drug that works amazingly fast to control bipolar mania.

After a week on the ward, I was visited by my life coach, and the ward allowed me to use the gym room. Back to training we went. I'm so incredibly grateful the staff allowed me this space to train and exercise again; it helped me massively. After three weeks sectioned, I was released from what felt like prison, and it was time to try and get back to life in the outside world. It was incredibly tough. I tried hitting the ground running – back to work flat-out, which didn't work, but I really wanted to put this episode behind me. The psychiatrist explained I needed a break, so I decided to take some time away from work and the stresses it brought. I had regular psychiatrist appointments where we discussed various topics, and I adjusted my medication dosage on several occasions. I asked for some of the antidepressants I'd used before – they had worked before; they could only help me again.

At first it turned into a nightmare. I experienced two episodes of elevated mood, the stage before psychotic mania. I took myself to A&E, with my mum explaining the situation to the on-call psychiatrist, who was shocked I was taking an antidepressant along with mood stabiliser drugs for bipolar. They gave me a second drug and my mood dropped to normal in ten minutes. After coming off the antidepressant, I got a different psychiatrist, and now I'm back on it but with a different mood stabiliser at a higher dosage. The second drug didn't sit right with me; I slept days away fighting depressive lows again till I got to crunch point. On the 19th of November 2020 I nearly took my own life. I planned to drive off the cliffs of Guernsey and end the pain. I was rock-bottom – life had beaten me.

From somewhere I found the strength to text a friend asking him to help me, and he literally turned up at my house half an hour later before I got in the car. He saved my life. He stayed with me for the day, and I then went to stay at my parents', booked the psychiatrist and opened up, explaining I couldn't take this drug any longer and I had planned to end my life. With my openness and talking, we decided to change my medication to another mood stabiliser, but it would take six months to do so. For this period, my legal high, Carlsberg, was out of the question, so I took a break from the booze and the parties and slowed life down.

Just over a year ago we received some tragic news. An old teammate and football friend had committed suicide. He had struggled with depression and had some issues none of us knew about, and, sadly, he ended his life. The island was shocked. Rest in peace, Scotty Bradford. It's so sad that he slipped through the radar – another tragic loss and trauma to add to my life experiences.

I was at a crossroads in life, stationary with no idea which way to turn. The break from work allowed me time to think about what I'd do next. I began volunteering, working as a peer support worker at the Oberlands Centre[1], helping others on their journey to recovery. As my stay in hospital had been so short, I didn't complete the ten-week recovery and well-being course as a patient, so I did it as a support worker, learning life skills I still use to this day. I got mental health first aid training along with SAGE & THYME Foundation Level training in dealing with distressed individuals, and I continue my work with Man Club supporting others. I set up a club in a secondary school, called Cloud9 Club, where I would openly share my journey and allow the young lads an opportunity to talk and be listened to. It was amazing; it gained traction and, through social media, donations were offered to support the project. After fourteen sessions with the lads, COVID kicked in and halted the progress of Cloud9. I was gutted.

In October 2022 I walked away from my business. After twenty years in the trade I'd lost my heart, desire and passion for gardening. I'm very much an all-or-nothing character. I can't be doing anything I'm not passionate about.

At the start of July, I put my dream house up for sale – I saw no other option but to sell the home I had worked so hard for, to get some money behind me as I had financial struggles and was in a little debt. Fortunately, I had met all mortgage payments. Accepting an offer on my house, reality hit me – "FUCK! I'm gonna sell up!!" Then suddenly the banks' interest rates changed, and the couple couldn't get the mortgage they needed. I believe to this day this was fate. The timing was wrong to sell. The next day a friend I met at Man Club checked in with me. "Checking in … how are you, Cockers?" I was open with him, honest about my financial position, my struggles, my latest battle in life. He said, "I've been in banking/mortgages all my life, and I want to help you. Shall I speak to your lender?" Wow, a possible breakthrough. I needed a break in payments basically, freeze my mortgage, add a year or so onto my contract. I stopped viewings on my house while I found my feet again mentally. The bank my mortgage is with is Skipton International. I've helped them with some mental health campaigns over the years. Due to my mental health, I was out of work and unable to make mortgage payments. Let's see if they really support mental health issues when they're met with mine.

In 2004 I'd qualified as a tree surgeon, and I most recently went self-employed as a tree surgery contractor, subcontracting out to other businesses. I'm able to work now, without the pressure of having my own company to run. On 1 January 2023, the company I was subcontracting for offered me a full-time contract. I took this opportunity and was loving my new position with work. During this period, a job came up at the Oberlands Centre's Adult Mental Health Service in Guernsey. The job title was "expert by experience", as they were searching for individuals with lived ill mental health experience after a review of the system highlighted a missing piece. This was a new role, so I was excited to apply. On the twenty-second of March I had my interview. On the same day they offered me the job. I'm so excited to get going with this new role and so proud of my achievement.

Unfortunately, after four to five months in total working for Arbology tree services, I hit physical and mental burnout. Depression fatigue is something very real to me. I took the chance to have a break from work and look after my mental health. I didn't feel right and was hit with a bout of depression where I couldn't think straight, I couldn't focus, and suicidal ideation would begin to kick in if I didn't escape my mind. So I slept ... sleep is like a reset of the brain for me and others. I checked out and slept for about two days, escaping my mind and the suicidal thoughts that had the potential to take over my brain. After this I began to feel slightly better and slowly build myself back up to my full potential. It takes time, though, and these episodes will hit me from time to time. I have great insight now into my illness; I know what I need to do.

I'm now filling out an application form to become a peer support worker at the Oberlands Centre in a twenty-five-hour-a-week paid role. I hope I'm successful. The hospital has been supportive in my application and combining the two roles, expert by experience and peer support worker in specialist mental health services.

I would like to be involved with as much mental health and well-being work as possible and hope I can secure both jobs at the

Oberlands, because helping others is where my passion is now. I hope it can be relatable to others who may be in difficult circumstances in their own lives. You can't coach, teach or get a qualification in life experience – but I've had many experiences. Together we are stronger!! Take care and keep talking!

---

1. https://www.gov.gg/oberlandscentreservice

REFLECTIONS

REFLECTIONS

REFLECTIONS

SIXTEEN

GRIEF: DAVE

Maybe you're like I was, thinking "leave school, get a job, a career, find a partner, have 2.4 kids and life will be pretty simple." As if it's on an uphill trajectory and in a straight line. Then, as you become more experienced in life, you realise life isn't like a straight line, it's more like a roller coaster, with peaks and troughs all over the place.

Life was great back in 2015. My training business was on course to have its most successful year ever, and my partner had found what she loved to do and was producing some amazing artwork. We had also been looking into the possibility of working with a couple of galleries to display her work.

Sounds great, right?

But if you'd been with me on the tenth of December 2015, you'd have been entering a white, square, clean-smelling room that was quite cool and kind of eerie. Covering about a third of the room was a blue sort of shower curtain.

I pulled back the curtain, and there she was. My partner, Helen, or "Hel" as I call her. Hel is about 5'10", with short brown hair and one of those grey streaks that runs from the front to the back of her hair that she absolutely despises. Hel is full of fun, a real joker, the yin to my yang, my rock, my world, my sparring partner. Hel is the love of my life.

"Mr Williams, it is now time for you to leave." It was the voice I didn't want to hear from an officious-looking doctor in a three-quarter-length white coat. You see, we were at the Royal Derby Hospital, and Hel wasn't being prepared for an operation; she was being prepared for the morgue.

For the next couple of months things went okay, because I was focussing on everyone else. I was supporting Hel's family, and indeed my own family, as anyone would do; but the reality was, I was distracting myself by focussing on everyone else. I was in denial, as I wasn't dealing with the things I needed to deal with in my life and so was delaying the inevitable. And I was questioning whether I was worthy, since I couldn't even look after my partner.

Being totally honest, I buried my head in the sand about everything I needed to deal with. I was struggling to get out of bed on a daily basis, and when I did, all I was doing was watching daytime TV. Well, I say I was watching; the reality was, the TV was on and I was staring at it, but I didn't really absorb anything that was going on. I was a bit like a moth in a trance, fixated on a light bulb. When I was talking on the phone to friends and family, I was putting a brave face on for the call to, hopefully, hide how I was feeling inside. Maybe you have done things like that?

In essence, I was just existing, and the reality was, I was totally rock bottom. Not only had I lost the love of my life, but I had pretty much lost my business as well, because I wasn't really functioning as a human being, even in my own company.

If you'd been with me on a February evening in 2016, you'd have been sat on my black sofa with white walls on either side and a red feature wall in front of you. I know the TV is in the right-hand corner and the bookcase is in the left-hand corner of the room, but on this particular evening I couldn't see them. The darkness I was feeling inside matched the darkness of the unlit room. The reality was, I was depressed, lost, lonely and wondering what the point of life was.

Have you ever felt like that?

I was listening to a lot of music that night which was very melancholic. Songs that resonated with me, songs that Hel and I used to listen to, or artists that I felt a real connection with. I just felt that I needed to have a connection to Hel and the better days that we'd had.

I was feeling so down, I hadn't really eaten that day. I had lost my confidence and really couldn't see a future for myself. All our plans had totally evaporated like a spell from a Harry Potter movie. In the days leading up to this night, I'd had constant thoughts of 'What is the point of going on?'

'Oh Hel, what am I going to do? What the hell can I do? What the hell is the point? Oh Hel, what would you say if you were here right now? Well, I guess you'd complain about the state of the room, for a start!'

'I could always jump off the bridge at the bottom of the road, onto the main road, which would be pretty quick, I guess. And you hear of people drinking themselves to death, don't you? The problem is, I'm not keen on alcohol. I guess it would be easier with a knife then, as no-one would find me for a while anyway.'

I honestly don't know what happened next, as it's all a blur. It may have been seconds or even minutes, I have no recollection at all. But the next thing I knew, I was standing over the kitchen units with a chef's knife across my wrists. That was scary and my "lightbulb moment", as I knew I needed to make a decision. Either to stay as I was, just existing rather than living (and I knew deep down I wouldn't be around much longer) or make the decision to change for the better.

Deep down, I knew I needed help, but I'm a guy, and guys don't ask for help, do they?

And if I had done the deed, whatever your beliefs about a greater force, I knew that Hel would have been so ashamed of me. Now that is a powerful bit of leverage to change! I went searching for answers to help me and tried a few things, but they didn't help me at all. So I started putting some strategies in place and found they began to have an impact for me.

Now, as soon as you decide to change and take action, life becomes a bed of roses, right?

Not necessarily.

On many occasions, I thought I had turned the corner, only to find another slide waiting for me to take me back a few steps. It seemed like my life was a piece on one big game of snakes and ladders, and I didn't have control of the dice.

Sound familiar?

But I kept on going, as my driver was *'What would Hel think of me?'* and to make her proud. She had left her impact on the people around her, and it was my time to grab hold of that baton and continue with her legacy, but in my name now.

I had to do a lot of soul searching, and being totally honest, it was very uncomfortable at times, and I really struggled.

Visualise this: feeling rock-bottom, emotionally numb, exhausted by putting a front on for others, trying to excavate positive things about myself, my life and what I could do moving forward to get my life back on track ... to stop just existing and start living again. In fact, being honest, I felt I had failed. Back to the snakes and ladders again!

But I knew this exercise needed doing; in fact, I decided it wasn't a need, it was something I *must* do. So I cheated! I put myself into what I imagined were Hel's shoes, and I imagined what she would say and do. You see, I was taking the emotional focus off myself and looking at the situation from a pretend third-party perspective. Imagine you're watching and enjoying a movie; you're watching from a third-party perspective where you can see what's going on but can't interact with it. Eureka!

This worked for me, and suddenly I could start to see things in a different light and started making notes like crazy of things I wanted to do for the future, whilst I was in that frame of mind. Okay, I ended up scribbling most of them out, *but it gave me a starting point*. The summary of my goals was printed out and stuck on my fridge so I could see them all the time.

Miraculously, my focus began to change, and I started to look forward instead of backwards. The way I'd been existing up to this point was like trying to move forward whilst staring in my rearview mirror, and the reality was, I crashed!

I was in such a bad frame of mind before my lightbulb moment. I had been talking to myself in such a poor way. It was very self-destructive; I just hadn't realised that at the time. Here's the thing – I was using the most negative letter in the alphabet for nearly everything; *T*. I was telling myself I *can'T* do this, and I *can'T* do that, etc.

Perhaps that's something you can relate to?

I have since summarised *CAN'T* as **Constantly Affirming Negative Talk**. Going through the aforementioned exercise, I had that epiphany and realised what I had been doing. No wonder I had been struggling!!

It was like trying to move forward wearing concrete slippers – pretty much impossible.

So I dropped the *T* and started communicating to myself what I *could* do instead of what I couldn't do ... and *can't* became *CAN*: **Confident Articulation Nails it!**

As I was starting to feel better, I started doing more. Instead of struggling to get out of bed daily and constantly listening to melancholy music, I began to emerge each day with more vigour and allowed myself to listen to more empowering, positive music. For me it was rock music with a good beat, and I also started exercising. It had been a while since I'd done any exercise, so my running was really slow, and I could only manage short distances initially ... I was so slow, I was being overtaken by snails! But little by little, this started to improve, and just like everything else I'd been doing, it was *progress over perfection*.

There were certain things that I was doing, but in the wrong way – so I shifted my thoughts and actions, and things started to get better. I started sharing some of these strategies I had created with other people, and found they were getting great results in a shorter space of time.

By chance, an email crossed my path with an opportunity to

become a qualified master coach. Hel and I had always been a magnet for others to come to and get their issues resolved, and it seemed a good, logical fit. And I now had something empowering to focus on. It felt like the light at the end of the tunnel.

As I was about to leave for the course in London, I got a massive bout of anxiety and decided to cancel. My inner demons were saying, *'Dave, how can you become a master coach when you can't even master yourself?'*

Have you experienced your inner demons talking you out of things?

I gave myself a good talking to (that's the polite version!) and rebooked the course, because my drive, my *must*, was stronger than my inner demons. It was a major milestone for me to get to London, and when I got there I had an issue getting out of the car. Those inner demons had travelled down with me, and it was so much easier just to start the engine and head home again. But I reminded myself of my *must* and made myself get out of the car and head into the event.

The event was held in a hotel by Heathrow Airport. The room was set up like a traditional training room. I sat right at the front, just in front of the stage, as I didn't want to miss a thing. The trainers started their presentations and announced that they were Tony Robbins (the world leader in life coaching) trainers. Just then a voice appeared in my head – not my inner demons this time, but my inner hero; in fact, it may even have been Hel – saying, *'See, you are in the right place.'*

Towards the end of the second day, one of the trainers, Nicky, approached me. How can I describe Nicky? She's a very glamorous, spiritual lady with blonde shoulder-length hair, wearing a blue and purple floaty dress – she wouldn't have looked out of place at Glastonbury.

"So then Dave, what's been the main learning from the course so far?"

"Well, I guess it's that so many people need help," I replied.

"Exactly, Dave, and with your experiences you know what people are going through and you can help them at a greater level than people who just learn from a book."

That was the beginning of my coaching journey, and I had my first client immediately. Funnily enough, this client was also depressed, had been focussing on the wrong things and generally not looking after themselves. Putting a brave face on for everyone else but deep down feeling awful.

You see, my very first client was *me*! I had to get myself right before I could serve others at an elevated level. I needed to be true and authentic so I could help others and not have my inner demons rear their heads again. Now, with the strategies I've learned from some of the best personal development leaders in the world, I'm able to show up and think, as the song from *The Greatest Showman* says, 'This is Me!'

So where do you find me now? You find me as a number-one bestselling author, multi-award-winning results coach and speaker who has had the pleasure of speaking and having clients on four continents around the world.

I'm helping businesses improve their profits and reduce staff turnover with The Management M.A.S.T.E.R.Y. University, and I have personal clients ranging from busy professionals and executives to police officers, athletes and single parents around the world, helping them overcome their challenges and start living life again instead of just existing.

You see, now that I've had those experiences, I'm better equipped to serve myself and my clients at a greater level, and life is great. I can now be more empathetic because of my experiences, although it was very painful at the time.

I have a wonderful partner and some incredibly special people in my life who enrich my life beyond measure. I'm so grateful to everyone who has been a part of my journey and helped me meet amazing people and experience wonderful things that I would never have considered possible a few years ago.

The great thing about life now is that I get the privilege of being able to impact others and enhance their lives through my coaching, training and speaking. This has impacted hundreds, if not thousands, of people around the world. This isn't supposed to sound like hyperbole by any means. I'm talking about the ripple effect. Everyone is having an impact on the people they interact with all the time, a bit like dropping a pebble in a pond and watching the ripples expand. Here's the thing: those ripples can be either empowering or disempowering. The people I have worked with have turned their ripples into empowering ones, affecting others in their lives.

I can only share this story with you because of making the decision to change, turning my situation from *wanting to change* to *"I must change."* My lightbulb moment was the catalyst. I had to reach my own pain threshold before I took that decision. If I hadn't had that moment, and made the right choice, you wouldn't be reading this, and no-one would ever have known my story because it would have stopped in 2016.

Has it been a journey with loads of peaks and troughs? Hell, yes! But this has helped me grow as a person and become a better person for it. In fact, it could be argued that I've had more comebacks than Frank Sinatra.

Now, obviously I don't know where you are on your journey, but I do know that you'll get hit by curveballs along the way. If you're facing challenges currently, then my heart goes out to you, but please remember that wherever you are, there is always a light at the end of the tunnel.

Will you make mistakes along your journey? Probably. We're all human and that's how we learn. If you make a mistake, don't worry about it. Focus on what you learn from it and make it better the next time. As Thomas Edison, inventor of the light bulb, once said, *"I haven't failed. I just found 10,000 ways that won't work."*

Always remember, you are a special, loved, unique individual who has already achieved so many amazing things in life. You have the opportunity to take your life to a better level and have a phenomenal life, positively impacting others around you. The world needs you and your unique experiences, qualities, and outlook.

Wherever you are on your journey, it is a chapter in your life, and the beauty of it is that you are in charge of the quill. If you don't like it, turn the page and write another chapter.

I'm sharing my story not as a "poor Dave" sob story – far from it. I'm sharing it out of love and respect for Hel, her family and the wonderful people who have impacted my life, both personally and professionally. You see, without the love of Hel, this story would never have been shared. I share my story with you from a place of love from Hel and myself to you, so you can see that wherever you are in life, things can always get better.

REFLECTIONS

REFLECTIONS

REFLECTIONS

SEVENTEEN

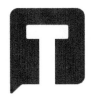

ABUSE: SAM

I'm almost thirty years of age and my life is getting on track after having a bit of a hard journey.

During my teenage years I got into drinking and drugs quite intensely. I started drinking when I was fifteen, started smoking cigarettes at the age of eleven, mainly because I was hanging out with nineteen-year-olds, and started smoking weed about the same age I started smoking cigarettes. I look back now and think, 'Why!?' but I know it was because I was hanging out with older kids.

At the age of eighteen I got involved in harder drugs due to the parties I went to, and it was only recently that I linked all the drink and drugs to events in my childhood.

Growing up in Spain with my mum and stepdad, we would always be going around to their friends' houses for parties and BBQs and everyday get-togethers. There were other kids there around my age (which was eleven), and I used to spend a lot of time with one of the boys in his room playing PlayStation. He was a couple of years older than me, so he was in a different place mentally, more mature.

Whilst we were in his room, he'd do things to me, and due to my age, I didn't realise that what was going on was as wrong as it was, but

I did know it was wrong. I know now that kids our age shouldn't have been doing those things. I don't remember how it all started, but he used me sexually to experiment with. It started out as touching and escalated to him having sex with me, whilst our parents were downstairs.

It was only when I was thirteen or fourteen that I realised what had been happening shouldn't have been happening. I didn't say anything at the time because I didn't want to upset the balance and friendships of our parents over something that they could potentially have said was nothing, but I know it was something – and something that should not have happened.

I know I should have said something, but as our parents were friends, I didn't want to cause any fallouts. It would happen every time we went around to their house, and so when I realised at the age of thirteen or fourteen that it was wrong and I didn't want it to happen anymore, I stopped going over to his house.

At fifteen I started drinking. In Spain it is a party kind of lifestyle, so the drinking started as a social thing and wanting to fit in. After a while I realised that it helped me to forget what had happened, and the more I realised I could forget, the more I drank.

I started going out with different friends, and then when I was sixteen, a friend of mine who was also sixteen was doing odd jobs for this older guy. We'd go out with my friend's boss, who was in his fifties, gay and married at the time. There was one occasion when we'd all had a lot to drink, and I ended up in this man's van with him, where stuff happened. I don't remember consenting, and it started to confuse me. I started to wonder if I was gay, so this was a really difficult time for me.

This was now the second time this had happened with a male, and I knew I never wanted it to happen again. I never said anything about what had happened with my friend's boss, other than to my friend at the time, so nothing was ever done about it.

It was only recently that I told my mum and stepdad what had happened, both with my friend's boss and when I was younger with their friend's son. They told me that I should have told them, because they could have done something about it, but again, due to my age I didn't know what could be done, or what would happen. I just knew I didn't want to upset the apple cart.

I've spent my adult life drinking and taking drugs to numb the memories and drown the demons. I would drink every weekend and smoke weed daily, which at the time was helping. During the parties, I would be introduced to other things which helped me to forget even more and helped me, I guess you could say, "enjoy life".

I found myself taking more and more drugs to forget and run from my past, and I realised that I couldn't keep running, which is why I ended up telling my mum and my stepdad.

As I had been abused by men both times, and I am attracted to women, it became a very confusing time. I haven't been able to stay present when I am with a woman; my past catches up with me and I freeze in the moment.

I've tried therapy, but because I get to a certain point, and we have to keep going over everything, I have got to the point where I have given up on therapy. I have been trying to cope with it myself by drinking and drugs, but as I am pushing thirty, I know I need to sort my life out and stop running, which is why I have now told my parents what's been happening; they are older and wiser, after all! I am hoping they will help me figure it all out.

I am weighing my options on how to move forward and see what kind of help there is out there for people in my situation. I know that speaking up is important so other people don't have to go through it alone like I did.

I've started going to the gym with my mum, as it gets me out of the house. I have spent a lot of time in the house by myself dwelling on things, which is no good for my mental health.

I am reconsidering therapy, a chance to speak with someone who is paid to listen and not pass judgement.

Speaking with my mum and stepdad was the first step in fixing my mental health, and it is this first step that is important. We can't fix our mental health by ourselves because it is incredibly difficult to fix it by ourselves. Accepting the fact that I needed help was quite hard for me, but once I had spoken with my parents, I did feel like a weight had been lifted. I'd been carrying this around with me for almost twenty years, and it was really starting to impact my life and relationships.

I do believe there was the stigma of having mental health issues, especially growing up around manly men, many who had the attitude of "just get on with it" and "be a man". In my head I believed they would think I was some kind of weirdo, wouldn't want to be around me and would tell me to get away from them. I never felt like if I had mentioned my issues, I would have been accepted. There was also the thought that they would think that if this had happened to me, would I now do it to them? The answer is mostly definitely no.

I would highly recommend that if anyone is going through something which gives them any doubt in their mind that what is happening shouldn't be happening, speak with someone straight away. If you think it is wrong, the chances are it probably *is* wrong. And make sure it is someone you trust and who has the power to help and guide you away from that situation.

For those who are using drink and drugs to mask or numb what is going on deep down, trying to run away from the memories, or as a coping mechanism, I'd suggest getting help for both the drinking and the drugs, as well as what happened in the past. One of the things I have realised is that even though the drink and the drugs were helping to numb the past, they were creating more problems for me. For example, all my parents saw was their son diving into drink and drugs for no reason at all, because they didn't know what had happened to me. I pushed my parents away and told them I needed to do this, but I never told them why. I pushed them away instead of pulling them closer. If I had spoken with them earlier, my life would have been very different.

When I eventually told my parents, their response was extremely positive towards me, which I think I knew deep down it would be, but

I also didn't think it would be. It could have gone either way. Looking back, I feel like an idiot for not telling my closest family about what happened, because why would they react badly to a member of their family reacting badly to something bad that had happened to him? I know, looking back, I was in a dark and grim place where everything looked different, but actually speaking out about it has allowed me to see the light at the end of the tunnel.

There was a little bit of embarrassment about speaking about this because it had happened to me, because you think 'it would never happen to me,' but it did happen to me; and I think the more we speak about it, the more we all realise that it does happen more than we think it does, and we can help prevent it happening to others.

No one wants to admit to themselves or to others that they are a victim or have been a victim, because there is a stigma around the word *victim*; and not just men, but women as well. It puts us in a bracket that we don't want to be in, and if we don't speak up about it, then we can't get the help we need.

REFLECTIONS

EIGHTEEN

FATHERHOOD: VIKASH

My name's Vikash, and I'm a bereaved father. I had my daughter on 13 October 2021. Her name was Jaanvi Lad, and she was with us for fifty-two days. Jaanvi got her angel wings a bit too early. This is the way my wife and I put it. We still don't know exactly what happened; the doctors are still investigating and trying to figure it out. They took blood samples from us and a biopsy from Jaanvi. All we know is at the time she had difficulty breathing.

I've been a civil engineer for ten years. I'm originally from Bradford but now am living in Birmingham, where I moved when I got married, to my best friend, in 2016. Things were going well; we'd bought a house together, got married and decided we wanted to start a family. The nesting phase we went through was busy, sorting out storage, getting the house ready, buying baby clothes.

The pregnancy wasn't the simplest; my wife suffered with something called polyhydramnios, which is excess fluid around the baby, but we were told it could be drained and was nothing to worry about. We were both understandably worried – my wife was only three months pregnant at the time, but she was so big she looked like she was six months. I remember trying to think of a reason she might have developed the condition. I was looking online, reading about other people's experiences. I did a lot of research, and I remember asking the doctor, "What can we do, what does it mean?" The doctor said that even with the scans, they couldn't determine exactly what the issue was. My wife, on the other hand, didn't do the same research as me. She wanted to know what was going on, but she took all her information solely from the doctors, rather than looking further into it and trying to come up with answers like I did.

When Jaanvi was born, she had trouble breathing. She spent the last few days of her fifty-two days on earth at a wonderful hospice called Acorns, who looked after us as well as Jaanvi, and helped us with all the arrangements once she'd left us. They're a wonderful charity; they're still helping us. They support both my wife and I with counselling, and one of the support workers still comes to see us after all this time.

When Jaanvi left us, things started to get difficult. We had to make funeral arrangements, getting her birth certificate and her death certificate at the same time, dealing with family and friends – people who often didn't know what to say and ended up saying the wrong thing at the wrong time. Nothing can make it better, but some things can make it worse, which you don't even realise until you're in that situation.

I wasn't planning on carrying Jaanvi's coffin. No-one should ever have to see a coffin of that size, let alone a parent, but my wife convinced me, and told me that this would be the last time we'd ever get to do anything for our daughter and that we should be the ones to do it. I remember my wife being distraught, whereas I felt very numb. Looking back now, I realise I had emotionally shut down, trying to be the man of the family, to be strong, a pillar of support for my wife. I don't think I showed any emotion on that day, it was just a day I needed to get through. All the people saying how sorry they were for our loss – I was numb to it, it just didn't mean anything.

After the funeral, we weren't sure what we should and shouldn't do. It was a very strange time. I decided to go back to work after a couple of months, which I realise now was the wrong decision. At the time, I thought it was the right thing: "just get on with it; it will be a distraction; I don't want to have to deal with these feelings." I think that going in to work actually magnified the emotions I was going through, which I really didn't expect – depression, anxiety, loneliness. I felt very lonely and like there was no-one else in the world that was carrying this weight, even though my wife had lost Jaanvi just like I had. My wife and I are both incredibly lucky that we drew a lot of strength from each other, and she's still my pillar of support.

I started suffering panic attacks. I would get butterflies in my stomach, heart beating a hundred miles a minute, at just the thought of stepping outside the house, let alone going to work and facing colleagues. And the sadness was always there; it hung over me like a black cloud, making me feel like nothing could ever get better.

Then someone from Acorns suggested that I talk to somebody, so I went to counselling through the Employee Assistance Programme at my wife's work. I talked to someone on the phone. We had about six hourly sessions. That first session, I didn't feel like it really helped. The counsellor was more of a sounding board, rather than giving me any tools to help. My wife then suggested that I try again with someone else, which I did. I had another six sessions with a different counsellor, and that did help more. She gave me some different techniques to try, a few imagery techniques, ways of being able to accept what had happened, and how to live with it. An analogy that I still remember was to imagine a ball in water, and to imagine that ball will sometimes sink to the bottom of the pool, and your life in the pool will carry on around it, and not be affected by the ball, but sometimes it will come up to the surface, and it will bob around and appear back in your life. This is the same as my emotions being triggered unexpectedly by a sight, a sound, a smell, a memory, some music – and then it's like being back at day one. I learned through the counselling that being able to express those emotions, being able to talk about it and let those feelings run their course, was a million times better than locking them away. It's always going to be there, for my whole life – that space that Jaanvi left in our lives is always going to be there, but we will have good days when the ball – the space that was left by Jaanvi – is right at the bottom of the pool, and more difficult days when it comes up to the surface.

After the counselling, I was still suffering a lot of sadness, and I remember my wife saying that I wasn't the same person I was before; a lot quieter, subdued, more in my own thoughts, I wouldn't talk to anyone. Even though I had these techniques to get over my emotions, I was struggling to connect with people and be able to engage with them.

My self-worth and confidence were really low, and the depression and anxiety were still there. I remember at one point, driving along the road, I had a fleeting – but very vivid – thought about what it would be like to crash the car, without hurting anyone else, but I'd be gone. Thankfully, when I asked myself, "Shall I do it?" the answer was, "No … because I have my wife, she needs me." She was the first person I thought of. I'd never had that kind of thought before, it had never crossed my mind, and it scared me. So I talked to my wife, and I talked to Acorns again. Acorns suggested I talk to someone from Sands, a befriender. As it turned out, he was also called Vikash, so maybe it was fate.

Vikash suggested I come along to the football group he went to every Friday. I told him I wasn't a footballer, I was useless, and he said that it wasn't really about the football, it just gave them all a chance to talk about loved ones who had passed on, and if I wanted to talk I could, and if I didn't, that was fine too. So I went along, and there were so many more people than I realised that had been through the same kind of thing as me. And I found out that every pregnancy has a 25 per cent chance of something going wrong, which I didn't know before. And all those bereaved fathers that were there at the football, they'd all been through something similar to me, and being able to talk openly and honestly about it, dipping in and out of everyday chat, and talking about our lost loved ones without worrying about what the other person was thinking or feeling, or whether they were finding it awkward, was a huge thing. We were all in it together. I didn't need to worry, because they'd all been through something similar.

One of my friends from the group put it really well: "This is the worst club to be a part of, for the worst reason, but it has the bravest, most courageous, strongest people that I've ever known." That's stuck with me because it's so true.

Being able to go to the football group and talk openly has helped immensely … and has helped me to be able to mention Jaanvi's name to friends and family, which was difficult to start with, because it made people feel awkward. We've also told them that it is okay for them to mention her name too, as it lets us know they haven't forgotten her. My wife and I talk to Jaanvi every day; we always sing her a little song at the time she was born, every day, and she's always with us, no matter what. But it really helps that other people are able to talk about her, to bring her into everyday conversation.

I've learned that being able to talk about my emotions, openly and honestly, without worrying about what the other person might be thinking of me, is so much more important than locking my feelings away, being a strong pillar of support, not showing any cracks in my armour. Doing that just eats away at us, and I think that fleeting thought of ending my own life would have gotten much worse if I'd carried on trying to keep my thoughts and feelings hidden away.

Thinking about where those values come from that I had previously – of being strong, being the provider, the pillar of support – I'd say from my parents, especially my father. My father came from India, got married to my mum in England and has worked hard all his life. He was the eldest of his siblings and so was expected to be the one to help the family. When he came to England, he felt he should provide for his family here as well as back in India, and this is where I get my values, my sense of what's right, what's wrong, what should be done, my duties and responsibilities – from him. He's a good man; he did everything that he was meant to do, expected to do in his life, but now I see that by always putting himself second in everything, he's got left behind, and that's made him a little bitter. And although I have the same values, I'd like to think that I've adapted a bit. I don't want to put myself second, because I want to be happy and content when I'm retired and playing with my grandkids, looking back on my life.

My values also come, to a certain extent, from my faith. I don't class myself as following any faith anymore, after what happened to Jaanvi, but before that I did call myself a Hindu and I was practising, on the path my parents set me on. In the past, my faith helped me in a lot of ways, with school, with work, and it instilled values and morals in me that I still follow now, even though I'm no longer a practising Hindu. Before Jaanvi was born, we conducted certain ceremonies and spiritual rituals that were meant to bring good luck and good health to the baby, so what happened to her broke that faith, that trust. I may turn back to my faith in the future, but not now.

Thankfully, I am in a better state of mind now. I've been off work for a couple of months, and I think that's played a huge part in my mental health improving, because I wasn't around the toxicity of a boss and colleagues not really understanding what I've been through and expecting me to just pick up where I left off, and not really realising that something like this fundamentally changes you, for life. *I didn't realise this either, before it happened to me.*

Our perspective, our priorities, our way of thinking, all change. Taking care of my family is still especially important to me, but I began to realise that looking after myself, and my mental health, and what makes me happy, is also important. It's not money, it's the simple pleasures in life – enjoying the sunshine, going for a walk. My way of thinking has been totally realigned by what happened to me. I realise I need to focus more on myself and worry less about trying to keep the people around me happy. I started to limit the circle of friends around me to those I knew would accept me at my worst, to also get me at my best. I now have people around me that I know genuinely care about me, who honestly ask me how I'm doing and really want to know the answer. Even though the number of people around me is less, they're the quality people that are left.

I'm in a better place now. I'm looking for work in my field and doing a delivery job in the meantime to pay the bills. It gives me a sense of purpose to know that I'm contributing to the household finances. I feel content after a good day's work, and like I've earned my weekends. It's a simpler job than what I was doing, but it keeps me busy. I've also got the confidence now to be more selective when I do decide to get a job in the field I'm trained in – I'll be more aware of the place, the people and the culture.

To keep prioritising my own mental health and the way I live now, I need to keep talking about Jaanvi, sharing her story with "anyone that will listen," as my wife puts it! My take on it is that I will tell her story to anyone that is worth sharing it with. Talking about her, and to her, really helps – we have photos of her dotted around the house. She would have been one year and seven months old now, and she's always with us. We each have her name tattooed on our chest.

If I could give any advice to another man suffering grief, I'd tell him, "Don't be hard on yourself", of which I'm my own worst critic. I berate myself. I tell myself off, and I blame myself for all kinds of things.

Remember, you're human, and you deserve as much empathy and understanding as anyone else. And you deserve to be able to get your emotions out. Just because you're a man, and we have this macho attitude of not talking about things and having a stiff upper lip and just getting on with it, you still need to get those emotions out and give yourself a chance to breathe.

The other thing I found is that, if you lose a loved one, you'll learn very quickly who your true friends are and who's really there for *you* rather than for what you can do for them. You'll be surprised who's there and who's not.

And most importantly, I'd tell you to talk to someone, not necessarily someone that can do anything about it, but someone that you care about and that cares about you. Lifting the weight off your shoulders by opening up is such an immense thing, and it does wonders for your heart and your soul. It works a lot better than you might think.

REFLECTIONS

REFLECTIONS

NINETEEN

ADDICTION: ROGER

I have worked in the city of Nottingham, England, for most of my life, and I've established myself in terms of working with lots of young people's initiatives, from criminal justice to mentoring. Occupational health and social care have been my background.

I've been serving the community in many ways, starting with door security in my early days, but a lot of that transformed into working with young people, early intervention and people coming out of the prison system through that revolving door – being able to offer them guidance in terms of fulfilling their dreams as opposed to going back to jail.

Over the years I've worked with drug addicts, the elderly, and people with dementia, Alzheimer's, Huntington's and Parkinson's, as I've always been a naturally caring person in terms of supporting others.

I was raised by my grandparents because my mum had me when she was sixteen, so she stayed with my grandparents during that time. By the time I got to the age of three my grandmother said to my mum, "Look, go live your life."

She met a guy who lived in Birmingham, so she went to live in

Birmingham and left me with my grandparents. They raised me from age three to sixteen. They were born in 1919 or 1920, and so a lot of the values I developed were very old school. By the time I'd got to the age of six or seven, I could clean my clothes; by the age of nine or ten I could iron my own clothes and scramble eggs and had learnt independence, which a lot of kids today don't develop.

They both worked very hard, which taught me to be able to be in a space where I didn't need to feel fearful. However, I did feel fearful, especially when the winter nights came. The dark became a big problem for me as I got into my early teens, but at the same time I learned how to be very independent. I got up and got to school. I didn't have anybody supporting me because my grandparents would leave the house at like 5:30 am, and I think that's where my getting up early in the morning came from. They never left me without breakfast; they'd wake me up at around 4:30 am and give me a bowl of porridge to make sure that I'd eat something before going to school.

I was brought up very much with a Christian belief, as was the way with the Windrush generation who came over. It was very much about big hats on a Sunday and going to church, and I remember being dragged by my grandmother to church twice on a Sunday, which was a nightmare.

By the time I got to fourteen, the rebellious side of me came out and I kept disappearing, not wanting to go. That quite quickly accelerated to when I was about sixteen and started to discover more about girls.

I think I took my own will back then, and basically I wanted to do things my way. I felt that my grandparents were too old for me; they weren't up to speed, trendy or wise. I remember being at a stage in my life where all my mates were wearing straight legged and I was still wearing bell-bottoms, wedge heels and platforms and was into the Bay City Rollers.

By seventeen I was living quite an unruly life, stopping out late, not coming back, not really listening. I had a girlfriend who got pregnant, and my son is now thirty-seven or thirty-eight. We could have had a life together, but it just didn't happen. I was really argumentative and challenged, as well as immature to the point where I just gave up and couldn't do it anymore. And I suppose I became this "walk", which is what an absent father was known as.

Around the same time, I started weight training and taking steroids, because it was the thing to do – everyone wanted to be big. It was the time for action star heroes, Bruce Willis, Sylvester Stallone, Schwarzenegger, and everything was about body image. And with that came becoming a doorman. I worked as a bouncer from the age of eighteen. I wanted to be in that environment because the people I looked up to, whom I saw as peers, were five or six years older than me.

Becoming a bouncer in those days was not like it is now. It was different because when the rave scene came along, all hell broke loose; it was ten thousand people in a field partying. I was naive enough to think this was exciting. I didn't really understand what came with it at the beginning, because we didn't finish till six o'clock in the morning. I remember someone saying to me, "Want to try a little bit of this?" It was this white substance, and I just licked it. It tasted disgusting, but within twenty minutes I was in a state of euphoria and couldn't stop talking. The music sounded brilliant, and I was wide awake, and I thought, 'Actually, this is quite good.' That was obviously the amphetamines, or "whizz", as it was known, which made me able to work and stay awake.

Then I remember someone saying to me, "Try these ecstasy tablets. Yeah, you've got to have one of these sometime." And it's funny because there was a movie called *Rise of the Footsoldier*, which is it a bit weird, and it portrays someone's first experience of taking a pill. And in it there was a song called "French Kiss", which was an amazing song, really kind of rhythmic. They had this lady's voice in the background, moaning and groaning, such a sexual thing. And I remember listening to that song whilst having my first experience of this ecstasy kicking in.

I remember my friends having one quarter of a pill just to see what it felt like. I took it as well and then said, "This is not really doing anything for me. Give us another bit more." They gave me another half and eventually I had a full one, and all of it came and hit me at the same time, and I thought I'd met God at that point. It was just such an unbelievable feeling. Anyway, obviously I fell in love with the mind-altering experience, which led me to moving to a place called Austria where I met my partner, who was a bodybuilder. She was light years ahead of me, great physique, she liked my humour and we got it on.

I went to Vienna, which was meant to be for six weeks, and she said, "Oh, I don't want you to leave. I really love you." And I thought, OK, and ended up spending the best part of twelve years in Vienna – a place where it's very, very hostile in terms of racism for every black face. I was in an environment where I knew nothing about the history, the very same streets where they took the Jews out of their properties.

I had to learn quickly that I was in a very hostile environment, and the one thing that kept me in a place of calm was knowing that I could come back to England and get involved with the rave scene. I knew I would be going back at some point and escaping all that negative racism and discrimination.

Things accelerated the bigger I got. Over a period of two years, I put on about four stone in size. I looked very intimidating. I was doing a lot of security work because I couldn't speak German. I refused to learn to speak German. Then a friend of mine over there said, "Look, I've got some work you can get involved in, close protection." And I was like, "OK", and he said, "Oh, you know, these are artists coming from America and you can spend some time with them." Again I said, "OK", to which he replied, "Just look after them." I turned up at this gig and got starstruck, because I was supporting and protecting Womack & Womack! Their big song at the time was "Teardrops", and I was like, "Wow!" And he said, "Look, just calm down, Rodge. Everything's good, man. Just make sure that no one gets to them."

I was a bit worried, but it was absolutely amazing. I'm this twenty-three-year-old and I just couldn't get my head round it, saying to myself, "It's real. I'm really doing this!" It really worked well for me, and then I had recommendations to support people like Tina Turner, David Michael Hasselhoff, Bros, Rick Astley, all these bands that were *huge* at the time. And then my greatest claim to fame was a manager in a band called Digital Underground, which at the time I'd never heard of.

There was this kid who was throwing popcorn at me whilst MTV were filming, and I remember someone said to me, "Oh, my God, do you know what who that was?" I said no. I just remembered this kid with long teeth throwing popcorn at me, and I'm stood there with my sunglasses on, big twenty-inch biceps creating this image, and it was none other than Tupac.

The reason I'm telling you this is because I'm from a small place in Nottingham called Santans. I'd gone to Vienna. I had no mentor, no support. Everything I was doing was by my own self. And then with all of that came the arrogance where my grandiose self-importance became something else. You know what I mean? Mix that in with a load of steroids and real childish, immature behaviour and you've got ego.

I became something else. I created this persona, and my reputation preceded me and all that kind of stuff. And then one day I came back to England, and I was asked to do some security.

One afternoon down at the Fountain pub, which was a notorious Nottingham Forest football fan pub, Newcastle United came to play at Nottingham.

I was enjoying the daytime incidents, and then the crowds started kicking off. I ended up with my head caved in with a hammer, which nearly killed me. That's when everything changed for me in terms of my level of vulnerability.

This incident put me in a place where people were looking at me differently. I got myself into a better place, and I wasn't the same Roger anymore. You've got to imagine my mindset. I was carrying all this muscle, there was no fear in me at all. And the one thing that I never relied on, or thought would ever happen to me, was somebody putting a hammer in my head.

Being put in a place where that level of vulnerability and anxiety started when I was around crowds led me to accelerated drug use. The only thing I knew to do was work on the door, do security. For a year I lost that ability, and in that year I isolated myself. That's when I came to realise that those people you think are going to be there for you, aren't. You realise you've entered a lonely world.

And with that realisation and isolation, I lost muscle size. I went from my eighteen and a half stone down to probably the best part of twelve stone, which was my true body size, and with that came body dysphoria, insecurity, not being valuable, not worthy enough. My reputation was gone out the window. The more drugs I was using, the harder it became to get back to who I was, and then I became dependent on them.

I remember accelerating, and I got to a place where I thought to myself, 'You know what? Let me try cocaine because I'm bored. I want something different.' I did that for a while, and I managed to have a job, which I held on to for some time, as a business manager. How I got that, I don't know, probably lied through my back teeth, but what I did was I realised that one of my assets was networking with people. I am a salesman, you know. I've had to learn all these skills and I managed to put this front on. I got a job, got married. I'd front for her all the time, ignoring if she needed to escape, and being in a place where I could just disappear from life and then come back.

I did that for a couple of years recreationally. It was the same time when everyone was wearing designer clothing. It was the machine, the Versace, the money, pennies, the yuppie era. The administration. I had a great time. It was really, really good fun, but it was all fake. It was all false.

Then I remember getting a phone call one morning from my cousin, saying that my grandfather had passed away, and I remember feeling numb. There wasn't a major impulse, because I was recreationally using narcotics, so the body wasn't in a place where I could feel that kind of emotion.

I went over to Jamaica, and we buried him. While I was in Jamaica, I was still using, and found more coke, better coke. Six weeks later, my grandmother passed away from a broken heart because she'd been married to him for over forty-five years, and that's when things got weird for me.

There was this feeling of such loss. It was almost like losing both my parents within a six-week window.

Back in England, I remember my grandfather's sister asking me, "How are you coping, Roger?" And I asked her, "Why did you say that?" to which she replied, "Because you've lost both your parents." It was like someone had hit me with a sledgehammer, a powerful realisation.

I don't remember going out, running out of drugs, or driving over Forest Road and finding a working girl I'd run out of coke, and I asked her, "Do you know where you can you get me some coke?" She said, "Yeah, of course I can." I told her to jump in, not even thinking in terms of police pulling me over or anything like that. I gave her some money, and I'm really surprised she even came back to me. She told me, "We'll go back to mine, and we can use it there." I agreed, and when we got back to hers, she came out and told me, "I need to be honest with you. I couldn't get any coke, but I've got some crack." I said to her, "Are you crazy? I'm not taking that!" She told me, "Listen, it's only once, you know. You won't get addicted to it. It doesn't work like that. People just say it to scare you."

So I tried it. And I'll tell you what, that first rock, it took me places. That was when my love affair with crack cocaine started. And with that, the degradation, the despair, the dishonesty, the breaking down of relationships, the people that I'd promised I wasn't going to do it again. I mean, it went on and on, and I went to detox in 2004.

In 2004 when I heard about the tsunami, I thought it was going to be life-changing, because I was hearing about all these hundreds of thousands of people who had died, and I was there feeling really sorry for myself that I was in detox. I came out and was told by the psychiatrist, "You haven't got an addiction problem. You'll be OK." And within twenty-four hours I was back on it. I was told I was all right.

I remember my last relapse. It was absolutely devastating. It was my wife that snapped me out of it all.

I was in the corner of the kitchen on the floor, crying, huddling like a little kid crying my eyes out, because the worst thing is when you're using but you don't want to use, and you've got no way of stopping yourself from using.

The panic sets in. You know you don't want to do this anymore. I was there creating a pipe and crying at the same time, "I don't want to do this to myself", but the pull is so severe and so hard that you're doing it anyway and crying at the same time.

And that's when my wife looked at me and said, "You're not the man that I married. I'm taking these children away. It's either you go get help or you'll never see us again."

I remember crying, crying crocodile tears of course, feeling sorry for myself, but at the same time thinking, 'How can I use?'

The drug is that powerful.

Within a couple of weeks, I had to move out the house because she was going to take the kids away from me. I ended up going to my mum's. I didn't talk to anybody for weeks, just stayed in the room. They were bringing food to me, drinks, running the bath. I'd have a bath, get out of the bath, eat, go back to bed. The shame was just so immense, you know. I had to sell my house, give my car back. I lost my job, obviously.

I was back to square one, back in my bedroom living at my real mum's house where I'd visited as a kid, and it wasn't easy. I didn't want to talk to anybody, and I stayed there for the best part of six months. Whilst I was there I had the opportunity to speak to a treatment centre in Derby.

I went through a whole assessment process, which was difficult because the arrogance in me at that point was saying, "I'm not going there. I'm too good for this and I'm going to be in there with all these heroin users. I've discussed all that stuff. I'm not anywhere near rock bottom."

And then there was even more of a rock bottom when I one day I was outside my mum's house and I started talking to this guy, and I said, "Oh, do you know where I can get crack from?" He replied, "I can get it for you." Bear in mind, my mum lives in the rural south of Birmingham, and two doors away from her house was a crack cocaine dealer. I mean, what are the chances of that?

The rampage started again, which was difficult. I remember going through my stepdad's jewellery box and finding a ring to spend on this shit, which I did, and the whole thing started again.

It was just total chaos again, until I found NA – Narcotics Anonymous – and started going to meetings. I couldn't get my head around what they were talking about. Everything I was listening to, it was like I felt I was better than all the others there, that I was more important than them. Sitting at my mum's one day, I remember thinking, 'You know what? I'm done. I can't do this anymore.' So I decided to take my life, because I couldn't do it anymore. That didn't work. I failed. But that feeling of shame and guilt just wouldn't leave, and eventually I attempted it again, and that attempt didn't work. Neither did the third attempt, and I thought to myself, 'You know what, I can't even get this right.'

Shortly after the third attempt, I had a phone call telling me, "We've got space for you in rehab. It's time for you to come." That was 21st June 2005.

Last week I celebrated 18 years of total abstinence. That place was the lifesaving catalyst for me *because* it was run by former drug addicts. The ones who'd got the T-shirt themselves, who were now competent and qualified therapists, support workers, and they help drive addicts through the process of finding recovery.

It wasn't easy. It was like being in a welcoming old car, which you're going to break down, this antique classic car which you take all these bits off of and rebuild with new bits. And a lot of it was very emotional. I was probably the biggest baby in treatment, because a lot of stuff was pointed out and nobody wants to have a look at themselves, let alone be accountable for anything. Your behaviours and the stuff that you did – you can't escape from what you did, but it's how you redeem yourself from it, and the ripple effect of practising spiritual values, love, compassion, empathy, and humility in particular.

It teaches you to become a more rounded person, and I made a decision to hand my life and my will over to the care of a God that I understood, and with that, the compulsion and obsession was done.

Surrendering left me with myself, and at that point I had to learn about me. You know, who's the real Roger? I put on all these masks over the years so that I didn't even know who I was or what I was, and I didn't even know that I didn't know myself. I had to learn to understand who I was and rebuild myself.

Through that process I've been able to help so many others in addiction. I became a drug counsellor, drug specialist, set up a mentoring interview. I went from drug addict to service manager for one of the biggest rehabs in Staffordshire, all in four years. That's for mentoring and an early intervention programme for young people to get them out of the life of drugs, crime, gang knife crime, County Lines[1] and sexual exploitation.

I've run that for twelve years and gained several accolades, including a Nottinghamshire Black Achievers Sports Hero award. I won the Points of Light award from the prime minister and had to go to Downing Street and collect my award. It meant a lot to me because, although it was awarded by David Cameron, who I'm not really a big fan of, he's the one who spoke to Barack Obama to get that award brought over from America, so it was endorsed by Barack Obama. And I can't imagine there will ever be another black president in my lifetime, so it was something very special to me.

All the important relationships that I fractured over the years have now been rebuilt. The only thing that really damages me is the fact that I'm still not seeing my children. It will be seventeen years this year. I would have liked for them to be at my side when I collected all my accolades and just be part of my life. To be honest, it's not even about the accolades, I just want them in my garden having a barbecue, watching football, and just talking about life in general. I've missed out on all of that because of the consequences of my actions, my behaviour.

My best thinking is what brought me to that place, and by the grace of God, I hope that one day that my children and I will meet. But however things turn out, for now I'm setting my stall out. I'm looking to be in a place where I'm running for election in 2027. I feel now, having worked for the community for that many years, having been an ambassador of the community, it's now time for me to look at changing things at a high level in terms of legislation and policy.

I've put in the groundwork; it's not me and my ego. This is people saying, "Roger, we can't get anybody more authentic than you." All my stuff's out there, so whatever political or, I don't know, spiritual warfare wants to come at me, then it's all out there already. I've got nothing to hide. Put me in a position where that level of transparency is needed and I'm not afraid of it. What I am afraid of, if I'm honest, is God. I got baptised in the middle of 2023, and I'm incredibly grateful that took place at church on Family Day. They filmed it, and the whole church praises, you know, over your baptism and wishes you all the best of success to walk in a righteous path.

I got engaged this year in the Maldives, a week before I got baptised, to my beautiful partner, who's a Christian as well. It's been difficult because everyone automatically thinks because you make this transition in your life in terms of being in recovery, you've recovered. But there's the other element, which is that the drugs and the alcohol are symptoms of what is underneath. It's about looking at your behaviour and changing your thinking and softening your heart.

Where I come from, men don't cry. I come from a place where, if you're cheeky, I'll fill you in. It was learned behaviour, although it's kind of primitive. I've come through that process, the ego and the alpha male characteristics.

I've worked in health and social care for over twenty years of my life, and I've realised that was never me. I'm a gentle soul, I'm a caring individual and I'm an empath. So it was like mixing water and oil. The powers of evil, if you like, dragged me along and I got sucked into a place where I wanted to fit in.

My whole life has always been about wanting to fit in, but now I know where my place is. My place is with God.

Before I ever got baptised, I was told, "There's an energy that's going to come in and try and drag you all over the place. It's not going to be happy, because you've been a loyal servant to that way of life, and suddenly now you're this new energy, this new power; the devil is losing you because you want to walk in a righteous path." It's almost like it was coming at me, because I had so much stuff trying to get me and then when I got baptised, it was like it grew steroids and was saying, "OK, you think you're going to get away from this? It's not going to happen that easily!"

One of the hardest things ever is the transition from the life you once had, and I thought being in recovery and practising spirituality were in that programme, but this is a different level now. This is a totally different level. I've redeemed myself of my sins, I believe that, but it doesn't want to let me go. It wants me back in, and I don't think I've ever experienced this within my recovery process.

Now that I'm reading scriptures and I'm really unravelling the onion of me, the real Roger, then I'm just a very gentle, sensitive soul. And there's a part of me that doesn't really want to let that go because it's been my protective mechanism for such a long time. It's just a slow releasing and baby steps and light from time to time. I do get into this place where I'm so spirit-centred and my heart is so open that I'm just crying tears of joy, tears of gratitude.

I've been a knife crime campaigner for sixteen years now, and I've been with mothers who have lost their children to knife crime. My award from the prime minister was for an event that we did called, *Taken Too Soon*, which was held at my football club, and police interceptors all came and played charity football matches to commiserate and celebrate the lives of those young people that have been murdered through youth violence.

I'm grateful that I'm in a place where I can support the community, to help others. It's a privileged environment, a privileged space to be in, because I shouldn't be here. I had my head caved in with a hammer; I should have been dead. I've overcome drug addiction, a drug overdose and suicide attempts, and I'm still there.

In terms of stigma or discrimination regarding my mental health struggles, when I was diagnosed as a crack cocaine addict, a lot of the sector staff that were recruited tended to be very middle class and white, so there was no cultural identification in terms of my ethnicity. What they would have on paper was a big black guy, a former bodybuilder, former doorman, who's a crack cocaine addict. That's what they would get as an assessment. I would then turn off, and there was no cultural identification.

When I got clean, I had help setting up a drug service with the support of the University of Central Lancashire and also the DATS, the Drug and Alcohol Action Team of Nottinghamshire. I got funding to set up as a culturally specific service working with black and South Asian people. It was called BAACIN, which stands for Black and Asian Cultural Identification Narcotic. When we filled in the documents to get the funding, we found that there were lots of key reasons why black and Asian people were not accessing drug treatment. The main thing that came up was the lack of cultural identification, along with being ostracised when you're in an environment where the therapist has no idea how to identify with you. It is very hard for people to open up to someone they cannot relate to.

There is also the mislabelling. A lot of black people and South Asian people, in terms of mental health, were mislabelled because the therapist didn't consider their faith or have a cultural understanding of how their brains work, or the implications of life as a black or South Asian person. When we look back to the 1970s, the incidence of misdiagnosis of black people and South Asian people is shocking. There were people with mental health issues who were never diagnosed, and because of a lack of knowledge, institutional workers gave the wrong medication to patients just to sedate them. And I experienced a psychiatrist telling me that I was OK, and as I mentioned earlier, within twenty-four hours I was back using.

No-one understood how crack cocaine affected black people, so when I got clean and I was studying, I contacted a guy called Aiden Grey, who's a crack cocaine specialist in the UK who spent plenty of time in Queens and Brooklyn trying to understand all the different conspiracies and theories around this particular drug. There is a theory that the CIA created this drug to suppress communities and then went further to medicate us because of our melanin. Crack cocaine in our system is much stronger and affects us differently than it does Caucasians.

As for what I would say to someone who finds themselves in situations like mine, there are two ways of looking at it. There's a part where people say to me, "If you hadn't gone through all this process, you wouldn't be the person that you are now." And they are correct, but if I had had the choice of doing a degree, a master's degree or a PhD, from the time that I was using, I'd be very, very highly qualified and it wouldn't have been painful; but it would have been more painful in terms of another level of sacrifice, not so severe in the emotional aspect. The loss wouldn't have been as big, but I would have put as much time and energy into studying as what I invested in using and abusing drugs.

The consequence of going through education and all that process is that there's an end result, which is going to be something that improves your life; it's not going to destroy your life and leave you with nothing. It's all about loss, you know? Do you want to progress in life?

Or do you want to lose everything that you've got – and it's not even the external stuff. We're talking about your self-dignity, your self-value, your self-worth your self-esteem, your family, your friends, your credit status, all of that. I've been fortunate. Out of all the people that come through treatment, in the world, abstinence is only about 3 per cent.[2]

And by abstinence, I mean there are many who claim, "Oh, I'm clean", but they're still smoking cigarettes. They're still having a drink. All they've done is decide to stop taking the drug of their choice. But I'm talking about true abstinence. I don't even take paracetamol. I have one coffee a day and that is enough to turn my head. My system is that clear, that clean; even coffee makes me giddy.

When you've lost your life, and you get an opportunity to live your life a second time round, you embrace it with both hands. I'm in a place where I'm just, I don't know, I can't explain it. I'm so confident. The best of times within myself, and a lot of that comes from regularly unravelling the defects of my character. It's like the peeling of an onion, and people from the outside are looking in. They'll always have a perception of what they think I am, but my friends, they know me. And I've got plenty of friends who love me, who know me, who know who I am, so I'm not really bothered about other people's opinions; that's the one thing I've learned, I suppose, coming through this process of personal development.

I've learned to redeem myself, and I think the biggest thing for me is learning to forgive myself as well.

---

1. A large widespread drug dealing operation across Britain
2. Source: The Fellowship of Narcotics Anonymous, NCA and DATS

REFLECTIONS

REFLECTIONS

REFLECTIONS

TWENTY

GRIEF: SHAUN

My journey with depression started an exceptionally long time ago. I'm now fifty-nine and I still suffer with depression and anxiety.

In the early 1980s I met my future wife on a blind date, when she was eighteen and I was twenty-one. I was not really looking for a long-term partner, as I was planning to head off round the world either on my BSA motorcycle or by any means possible. But we hit it off, and Hayley quite liked the idea of some time travelling the world before settling down to a normal life, normal job, etc.

Sadly, not long into our relationship, her beloved father, Norman, succumbed to cancer after a short battle, and Hayley took it quite badly. This was the trigger for her lifelong battle with depression that I supported her through – and it also put a stop on our plans of world travel, as the bouts of depression could at times be so all-consuming that just existing was a full-time job.

Our path was not an easy one for a variety of reasons, but one of the hardest to deal with was that when Hayley got low, she would go on a spending spree. I didn't have a clue this was happening, and I'd find out just before the sh*t hit the fan. This happened on two occasions, but I was extremely lucky to be working in a job where overtime was almost limitless with very few restrictions. With a little juggling I managed to keep all the balls in the air, but this started to take its toll on me, as I was working six, sometimes seven days a week for usually fourteen–sixteen hours most days, and then trying my hardest to spend what little time I had left with Hayley. Looking back, I have no idea how I achieved this and when I slept!

My first experience of anxiety was after a particularly nasty lorry crash at work and my realisation that everything we had depended on me keeping it all together – my life was like a house of cards, and I was the major support. If anything happened to me, then who would be patient and caring enough to support Hayley, and who would keep the house payments going, as I was convinced that without my support Hayley would struggle. I had witnessed those crashing low points enough to have grounds for worry.

This pattern went on until my late forties. I was worn out physically and mentally, and the anxiety was becoming more of a problem. After the accident, I'd undergone over a year of weekly counselling meetings funded by work, but the anxiety still nibbled away at me. I had to reduce the hours I was working for my health's sake, but this also meant a reduction in the amount of money coming in.

Hayley had always worked, though at times she would be unable to leave the house and was often physically sick because of her depression. This did result in job losses, but she always went out and got another job once she was back on her feet. She never gave up and neither did I, but the pressure was always on me to keep everything afloat.

Then in mid-2012 Hayley dropped the bombshell that she had done it again for the third time and accumulated another massive debt! Only this time I was not able to bail her out. I had already maxed out the amount I could borrow on the mortgage and had an overdraft of nearly £20,000. *But* – and the memory sticks in my mind to this day – she sat me down and said that this time she was going to sort it herself and had been in contact with an agency that helps you manage debt. For the first time in oh, so many years, I saw the confident, happy Hayley that I'd fallen in love with all those years ago.

Those next few months were some of the best we had had in over twenty-eight years together. I was working fewer hours and we had even started to plan our escape. I'm a postman and can take my pension at fifty-five, so we were going to sell up once I'd reached retirement age. With the money from the house and my pension pot, we were going to move to France, a country we both had fallen in love with. Hayley would get her farmhouse where she could start her shabby chic business, and I would finally get my workshop for building vintage bikes and start a small vineyard. Finally, life was looking up.

But – and isn't there always a 'but'? – this was not to be. On the evening of 3 January 2013, I went to bed around 8:00 pm, as I had a very early start the next day, and I left Hayley downstairs watching TV. I was awakened by a strange noise downstairs. Assuming Hayley had fallen asleep, I rolled over, then thought, 'No I'll go down and wake her up.' I came down the stairs to find her flat-out by the back door, making the most awful guttural breathing sound I have ever heard. I tried to get her comfortable, then I dialed 999 and had an ambulance there within minutes. They tried to get her to respond but failed, so she was "blue-lighted" to hospital. At the hospital it soon became apparent that Hayley had suffered a massive burst aneurism, and the cognitive side of the brain had been crushed and it was the primal side that was keeping her breathing (I may well have these facts wrong, as I was struggling to comprehend what was being told to me).

From about 1:30 am I sat alone with her until around 6:00 am, when I knew my mum would be up. I got the nurse to ring my parents to let them know what was happening. I didn't want to disturb anyone too early, as there was nothing anyone could do. The next few days were a blur, and a lot happened, but she was finally moved from the critical unit to a room where she could pass peacefully. I sat with her holding her hand until she breathed her last breath in the early hours of the sixth of January, and then I went home alone.

Little did I know that my problems (mentally) were just starting. I don't know whether it was the shock of the speed of Hayley's passing or the fact that for all those years I had stood strong for Hayley, not allowing myself to waver, but I crashed, and I crashed badly!!

Not immediately; it kind of sneaked up on me.

I'd been doing a dry January, and I kept to it, apart from on the day of Hayley's funeral when I had a couple of brandies to steel my nerves. I made it into early February before I started binge drinking. I wasn't working, as I needed time to get my head together, so this left me in the house alone with whiskey and wine, and boy did I cane both!

I was extremely lucky to have some good friends who looked out for me, including one who phoned me on Valentine's Day to help ease the pain – cheers, Phil! But those hours alone with just my thoughts almost became too much.

The doctors put me on medication for my anxiety attacks, tweaking the dosage to help with the growing depression, but the lows kept coming. I was sleeping on the sofa as I could not face the bed alone, and I was swinging from days of being sober with no alcohol to drinking a bottle of whiskey in a sitting.

At this time, the only things keeping me from curling up and fading away were the constant support of my friends, real and virtual, and the pair of rabbits Hayley and I had. They needed feeding and keeping clean, and they became my focus in those early days, but nothing was pulling me from the gloom until I visited a local animal rescue centre with my parents on the pretext of getting them another dog. Only it was me that found a dog, and this is how Harvey came into my life.

I got Harvey for a couple of reasons.

One: I like road trips and planned on driving down to friends in France, so I fancied a travelling companion.

Two: There had always been dogs in my parents' home, and I felt that one in mine could maybe make all the difference. As they need walking, it would force me out of the house, which, thankfully, it did.

Getting Harvey was the turning point for me, and he became my constant companion. My parents and I had a time-share arrangement where he lived with me but when I was at work he was with them, so they got their daily walks, but they didn't have the responsibility of him full time.

We went everywhere together, and he slipped into my life like a well-worn glove, but the low days kept coming. I can recall three occasions where I woke up in the night, went to the kitchen and pulled out the bottles of paracetamol and a bottle of whiskey, and sat at the kitchen table with tears streaming down my face and that feeling of hopelessness that I have never been able to really describe. With one thought on my mind, and that was to end it. Only to hear a sound nearby, and I would look round to see Harvey emerge from the darkness and sit and look at me with his wagging tail and that grin he had.

The first two times, I closed the pill bottle and put away the whiskey, gave him a cuddle and went back to bed. But on the third occasion I dumped the pills and poured the whiskey down the sink!

I'd come oh, so close to pulling the plug on those days, and I am convinced that if Harvey had not been there the results would have been hugely different.

Then, in early February 2014, I woke up one morning on the sofa with a feeling that life needed to move on.

A good friend had told me that I needed to move forward and live my best life in Hayley's honour, and that if I just wasted my time, that would be two lives lost … and I had that choice and Hayley didn't.

At the time I didn't want to hear it, but she was right, and it was the kick up the backside I needed.

On that very same morning I decided that the pills I was taking were not helping me but just keeping me in the status quo, so I went cold-turkey. To move forward I needed to *feel* again, and the medication just made me numb.

Now in hindsight it was not a very sensible move, and it is not something I would recommend anyone else trying (please, if you feel your medication is not right for you, talk to the professionals) but for me it worked; I felt rubbish for a few days, but I then felt alive again.

A couple of days after my cold-turkey experience, I was asked along to a workmate's birthday drinks by a female work colleague. The day arrived and it was torrential rain, Harvey was spending the night at my parents', and I very nearly didn't go.

This would be my first social engagement on my own since losing Hayley. I'd been to car shows and events but always in the company of good friends, and I was terrified! So I did the obvious thing. I booked a taxi and asked the female colleague if she would like a lift, my reasoning being I would be less likely to back out if I had company. It had never occurred to me that my colleague was testing the waters to see if I was ready to start dating again – hence the invite. Up until this point I had had no intention of starting another relationship, and I fully intended my future to be just Harvey, Bruce, Cookie (the rabbits) and me.

The evening was a success, and I walked Claire home. We talked nonstop, and it turned out to be the start of a whole new chapter in my life.

Was I ready to start again?

I very much doubt it, but I also wasn't ready to stop living, and what did I have to lose?

Our relationship blossomed, but it also threw up issues I had never expected. I found myself confused as I was struggling to love two women at the same time. I felt I was being disloyal to Hayley by sharing my time with someone else, and I was also feeling like I was cheating on Claire with my love for Hayley. Irrational thoughts, but when you tend to overthink things, it is amazing what your mind throws up.

I carried on as best I could, keeping it to myself, as I am fully aware of the strain that living with a depressive can put you under. Another big challenge was when Claire mentioned that she would really like a child, and if that were not my thing then I needed to be aware that maybe our relationship wouldn't work out.

Neither Hayley nor I had wanted children, and I wasn't convinced that would change, but I remember sitting at home alone with Harvey and asking him what I should do. After loads of thought and much indecision, I decided to throw my dice and see where they landed. If it was meant to be it would happen; if not, nothing had been lost!

Of course, it didn't take long for Claire to fall pregnant, and we planned for the arrival of "Bean", as we didn't know the sex of our little one. I still was not sure about the direction my life was taking, but I was willing to give it a go. This period was stable for me apart from the constant battle in my head over loyalty to my two loves.

Our daughter, Poppy, was born on 22nd February 2015, and the feeling I got watching her being born only a stone's throw away from where I had watched another life slip away only a brief time ago was indescribable! I slipped into family life far quicker than I expected, and having this child really changed how I perceived the world.

But there was always this blackness in the background, and it was starting to eat away at me again, getting stronger and harder to deal with.

I finally succumbed and spoke with my doctor, fully expecting them to put me back on medication – but instead they pointed me in the direction of Cruse[1], the bereavement counselling service.

I'd been told of this service by a good friend but had failed to follow it up.

Finally, I plucked up the courage to call. One of the hang-ups I have with my anxiety and depression is my problem talking to people on the phone or even asking close friends for help. I really need to build myself up and I tend to function better when pushed into a corner, because then my hidden inner strength comes to the fore!

I started one-to-one counselling with the most excellent counsellor, who had the knack of saying very little but extracting volumes from me that even I didn't know was there.

It took a year of fortnightly visits before I was finally able to lay my late wife's memory to rest and start to enjoy the here and now. I have learnt that what we do and feel now does not detract from what we felt in the past. I walked away from those sessions a changed person in some respects, but still there was something lurking in the darkness.

Low days appeared with feelings of hopelessness and helplessness, even though regardless of all that had happened in my past, I was in the best possible position I could be. I had a wonderful partner, a daughter I could not love any more than I do, my faithful sidekick Harvey the hot rod hound, money in the bank and a shed full of old vintage motorcycles and cars.

You could say I had it all, but still the darkness would descend, and I would struggle to leave the house and go to work. I would look around and think, 'What's the point?'

On Christmas Eve 2018, my mum passed away after a short battle with cancer, so life switched up a step as my brother, sister and I had to care for our widowed ninety-three-year-old dad.

Again, having to look out for someone else took over that part of my mind that was usually awash with random and often damaging thoughts, and the following year was a solid and stable one for me. I did have my lows, but nothing to be concerned about, and then in early January 2020 on exactly the same date as I had lost Hayley, my dad passed away after a short spell in hospital, and that is when I took a nosedive back into deep depression.

I was unable to function for a couple of weeks as I processed the loss of both my dad and, of course, my mum, who I had been unable to mourn because of caring for Dad.

So again, I took the decision to speak to someone … and then COVID hit. My partner and I were both considered "essential workers," so our lives carried on as normal whilst all around us the world fell apart.

I started online and telephone counselling and began to study cognitive behavioural therapy (CBT), learning how to interpret thoughts differently, and the small exercises really started to help. It didn't cure anything; the lows kept coming, but I could manage them and keep myself buoyant.

Sadly, 2020 proved to be a tough year as I lost seven close friends and work colleagues to a variety of things including COVID, RTAs and suicide ... but all through this I kept an even keel and was managing well. Then a friend named Grizz came to visit me in between lockdowns. We drank tea, talked the usual rubbish, and made plans to build and race our old vehicles at various events once all the madness had subsided.

That was the last time we got to talk. He was diagnosed with an aggressive brain tumour a couple of weeks later, and he declined quickly and passed away in May 2021. I took his passing very badly and took another nosedive into the blackness, when I suffered with negative self-image and a real lack of self-belief and confidence, and when the friendship of someone like Grizz – who didn't suffer fools – would have meant so much.

The one thing that kept me going, kept me pushing forward, was the knowledge that no matter how dreadful things got, Hayley never ever gave up, so neither would I.

Once I'd put this episode behind me – and it took a few weeks before I could face the world properly – I continued using my CBT skills to minimise the effects of my mood swings.

Things were going well for me; I'd get the lows, but I was finding I could spin them round quickly by thinking of something positive. I am incredibly lucky that my work patterns mean I can walk my daughter to school every morning, and those walks where we talk, and she points out things that catch her eye, have made such a difference to me. Poppy has opened my eyes to the little things that used to thrill me as a child, and reconnecting with nature like we have has been such a joy!

The year 2022 arrived and it was not the greatest of starts for me. My chronic glaucoma had started to become an issue, and I was awaiting a hospital appointment. I also started the year barely able to walk, as my back had seized up, and it took five weeks of little activity and a course of anti-inflammatory pills (which caused other issues) before I was able to return to work.

In May 2022, the worst thing that could happen, happened: my beloved Harvey developed lumps on his neck. At first the vet thought it was an infection, but I knew in my heart what it was, and when after a week of medication things had not changed, they took a biopsy of the lump, which confirmed he had an aggressive form of lymphoma. He was given around four to six weeks to live, without treatment. The result being that on the ninth of June I had to take my boy for his last visit to the vet. An incredibly good mate drove me there and home again so I wouldn't be alone, as my partner was unable to get the time off work.

Losing Harvey triggered the biggest crash I've had since losing my wife. I didn't take much time off work because of the weeks I'd spent sick at the start of the year, but I'm not sure that was a clever idea!

Harvey's passing coincided with the discovery that I had suspected prostate cancer after a blood test for something unrelated; the doctor decided to do a PSA test only because I was over fifty, and man, am I so glad she did.

It was confirmed via a scan that I had an abnormality on my prostate, and I was booked in for a biopsy. Now, as I've mentioned, I tend to overthink things, and I started thinking about the connection between my bad back, the diverticulitis symptoms I was experiencing (caused by the anti-inflammatory meds) and the cancer. I added 1+1+1 and it came to 52 … and I was convinced it was all related and that the back pain and side discomfort were all part of the cancer and that I was on borrowed time!

I was scared shitless, but I told no one. I kept it inside. I'd walk to school with Poppy with a smile on my face and a spring in my step, whilst inside I would be asking myself, "How many more of these walks am I going to get?" Couple this with how I was feeling about losing my best mate and constant companion Harvey, and I could not get any lower. But outwardly I doubt many would have known of my turmoil.

I'm happy to say that the glaucoma worry has receded and is no longer a pressing concern. Yes, I do have prostate cancer, quite a bit in fact, but it is the lowest-grade cancer there is, and they're happy to monitor me and take no immediate action. And the back problem and side discomfort were in no way related to the cancer.

But all of this has left me in a hole I am struggling to get out of, and I'm back talking with a counsellor who is every bit as good as the lady from Cruse was all those years ago. I was looking for answers as to why I get the way I do. I had hoped that if I knew the source, I'd be able to control the problem, but currently I'm not so sure! The past is the past and I have no control over that, but what I do have is the chance to change today and therefore shape myself a better tomorrow.

What have I learnt from my journey so far?

I've learnt from Hayley that no matter how bad it gets, tomorrow will hopefully be better, so you need to be there to see it. Talk to people; do not keep it inside, as it becomes toxic and all-consuming. Think positive as much as you can. I've run a little experiment lately where I've noted what happens around me whilst in a negative mood and the day feels like crap, and then I've also taken note to see if the same happens when you're in a good place and the day is going well … and my conclusion is that the same things happen day in and day out, but it's your mindset that controls the day. Negative really does breed negative! And for me, writing my thoughts down has been a godsend; getting them out of my head and out into the world really does ease the burden.

I'll leave you with a thought, and it is this:

Despite what your head tells you, you're not alone in this.

Reach out and you'll be surprised who around you are the same.

I've often thought of my life in terms of surfing. You enter the sea and learn to stand up; as you go you get better and better until you are proficient at it, and then, BAM! a wave takes you out. Whether you were overconfident, or it was a rogue wave, it matters not a jot! You're under the water fighting for your life, and you finally break the surface and retrieve your board; you now have a choice about whether to paddle back out and get ready for the next wave, or turn to the beach and give up!

I've chosen to paddle back out. I know at times that paddle-out will be damn hard, but the ride is fully worth the effort.

―――――――――――――――――

1. https://www.cruse.org.uk/

REFLECTIONS

REFLECTIONS

GRATITUDE

Firstly, I must extend my deepest gratitude to Becks. Your unwavering love and patience have not only supported me personally but also fueled the creation of #MANUP and Tough To Talk. Without you, these stories may have remained untold.

To the steadfast pillars of the Tough To Talk trustee board - Eryn, Stuart, Tim, and Simon, your constant support and counsel have been invaluable. You've kept the mission at the forefront, providing guidance when needed, and for that, I am eternally grateful.

Our publisher, Dawn, deserves a special mention. Your patience is infinite, your passion contagious, and you've been our rock throughout the journey of creating #MANUP. Your dedication is truly appreciated.

Lastly, but by no means least, we must remember the men who have bravely shared their stories. By opening up about their journeys, they have shown all men that they are not alone. They've demonstrated that vulnerability is not a weakness, but one of the greatest tools in embracing true masculinity. Their courage is a beacon for us all.

DAWN PUBLISHING
ARE YOU A WRITER? DO YOU WANT TO GET PUBLISHED?

Then make sure you visit our Author Academy and check out our author courses, manuscript assessment services and 1:1 coaching with our award winning, international bestselling and founder Dawn Bates

https://dawnbates.com/writers

See how Dawn can help you on your journey to becoming published!

To discover more about Dawn Bates and her latest book releases, competitions and offers make sure you sign up for her regular weekly-ish emails using

https://dawnbates.com/dive-in

Printed in Great Britain
by Amazon

45763138R00169